PRAISE FOR

Innovative Staffing for the Medical Practice

"Deborah Walker Keegan has again captured the essence of the ever-evolving medical practice environment. In her new publication, *Innovative Staffing for the Medical Practice,* Dr. Keegan presents a timely and relevant resource… that is a must for the administrator's bookshelf. [Her] innovative approach to staffing models is demonstrated in her presentation of high-performance care teams, virtual patient flow models, virtual medicine, and accountable care. [She] goes to great lengths to present new methods of streamlining the patient experience, and giving patients what they want, when they want it, as being a must/prerequisite for consideration when developing an efficient staffing model for medical group practices.

Deborah Walker Keegan has hit the mark with another excellent book which is relevant, timely, innovative and, as always, very well-written."

DARRELL L. SCHRYVER, DPA
Chief Executive Officer
SOUTHERN CALIFORNIA ORTHOPEDIC INSTITUTE

ॐ

"*Innovative Staffing for the Medical Practice* is an invaluable resource for senior executives and administrators tasked with creating staffing teams to effectively manage the needs of the patient across a broad range of delivery systems. It is a very comprehensive tool, addressing all functions of a medical practice, and ultimately sets a new standard for the analysis, development, and deployment of staffing strategies, now and in the future.

Now, more than ever, a 'service-oriented' public is expecting value for [its] healthcare dollar. The ability of our healthcare 'teams' to manage the expectations of patients, payers, and government regulators can be both rewarding and challenging. *Innovative Staffing for the Medical Practice* is the necessary resource for medical practice operations."

PATRICIA L. BREWSTER, MHA, FACMPE
Chief Executive Officer/Partner
INTRAHEALTH GROUP

ॐ

More praise …

"In our work as medical practice consultants we regularly receive calls requesting assistance with staffing issues. In this book, Deborah Walker Keegan clearly presents tools and options for every medical practice to use in evaluating its staffing needs and developing optimal staffing plans. The chapters are filled with useful tips and clear insights into the changing world of medical practices.

I am particularly struck by the observation that as we move into the future of healthcare, it will be necessary to reorganize our staffing from a plan that is built around supporting the physician to one that is patient focused. This change will necessitate the building of care teams with new alignments of skills.

This book explains how the practice manager of the future will be competent in adapting staffing to the unique and specific needs of each work session. This is an essential textbook for every medical practice executive."

THOMAS H. STEARNS, FACMPE
VP Medical Practice Services
STATE VOLUNTEER MUTUAL INSURANCE COMPANY

ॐ

"During these economic times...this book is an informative and most timely tool. Management must be continuously cognizant of...staffing levels and the consequences of inadequate and inappropriate staffing and the effects it can have on the medical practice.

Now is the ideal time for all medical practices to consider innovating staffing in all areas of their practice.

Dr. Keegan's most recent book *Innovative Staff for the Medical Practice* will prove to be an effective tool for management during these complex times and...continue to be beneficial for many years in the future. The 'Staff Benchmarking Process' mentioned in her book is a brilliant tool in which to establish the appropriate staffing needs of the practice."

DONNA P. STEINMETZ, MSHA, FACMPE
Chief Administrative Officer
UNIVERSITY OF CALIFORNIA, IRVINE
DEPARTMENT OF SURGERY & NEUROLOGICAL SURGERY

ॐ

"As a healthcare executive for more than 20 years, the many changes in the patient care and the medical practice management world have been phenomenal...With reductions in reimbursement, more regulations than ever before, higher customer expectations, and a need to see the edge of success in our every day, I am always hungry for innovative strategies to assist me in leading my various medical practices and physicians to optimal outcomes, then leading to balanced practice standards and satisfied customers and staff.

The concepts, strategies, and benchmarking tools provided in *Innovative Staffing for the Medical Practice* by Deborah Walker Keegan provide all the nuts and bolts we, as leaders, need every day to be successful. Knowing Dr. Keegan as a past consultant in my medical practices, I respectfully stand up and take notice when [she] provides tools for success in the world I relate to. ... I thank you for this resource."

PAM SCHNEIDER RN, MSN
Executive Director/Administrator
OUTPATIENT CLINICS
LODI MEMORIAL HOSPITAL ASSOCIATION, INC.

Tina,

Thank you so much for your support! Innovate your staff model I have faith!

Deborah Kerigan

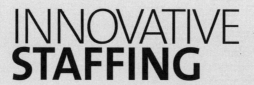

INNOVATIVE
STAFFING
for the Medical Practice

Deborah Walker Keegan
PhD, FACMPE

Medical Group Management Association
104 Inverness Terrace East
Englewood, CO 80112-5306
877.275.6462
mgma.com

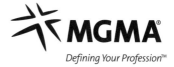

Production Credits
Publisher/Senior Content Manager: Marilee E. Aust
Editorial and Production Manager: Anne Serrano, MA
Copy Editor: Mary Kay Kozyra
Compositor: Virginia Howe
Proofreader: Katharine Dvorak
Indexer: Sara Lynn Eastler
Cover Design: Amy Kenreich and Brittany Hass, Studio Pattern

Library of Congress Cataloging-in-Publication Data

Keegan, Deborah Walker.
 Innovative staffing for the medical practice / Deborah Walker Keegan.
   p. ; cm.
 Includes bibliographical references and index.
 Summary: "This book offers tools and techniques to help medical practice administrators create the "right" care team for their medical practice--one that is current with today's delivery system and that optimizes provider productivity and efficiency, practice profitability, staff recruitment and retention, and patient value"--Provided by publisher.
 ISBN 978-1-56829-382-0
 1. Medicine--Practice. 2. Personnel management. 3. Medical offices--Management. I. Medical Group Management Association. II. Title.
 [DNLM: 1. Personnel Management--methods. 2. Practice Management, Medical. W 80]
 R728.K439 2011
 610.68--dc22
                        2011000717
 Item 8262
 ISBN: 978-1-56829-382-0

Printed in the United States of America
10 9 8 7 6 5 4 3 2 1

This book is dedicated to my husband, Mike. Thank you for your constant support and unconditional love.

I also want to acknowledge three of my friends and colleagues who freely share their talent and expertise with me:

- Elizabeth Woodcock, an expert in patient flow and all things data;
- Fritz Wenzel, a gentle man and teacher extraordinaire; and
- Marc West, a brilliant mind who encourages others to be their "best selves."

I am forever grateful.

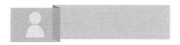

About the Author

Deborah Walker Keegan, PhD, FACMPE, is a nationally recognized consultant, keynote speaker, and author. She is known for her dynamic, educational, and high-energy presentation style, and her seminars and books are rich with "real-life" case material to enhance learning. They are packed full of tools and techniques that are relevant and practical for today's healthcare environment.

Dr. Keegan is President of Medical Practice Dimensions, Inc., and a Principal with Woodcock & Walker Consulting. With more than 25 years of experience as a medical practice executive and healthcare consultant, she assists clients in resolving a wide range of challenges facing healthcare organizations today. Her consulting services are in demand by hospitals, integrated delivery systems, private medical practices, and academic practices alike.

Key areas of expertise include:

- ➤ Practice operations assessments
- ➤ Revenue cycle assessments
- ➤ Physician-hospital integration
- ➤ Physician compensation plan redesign
- ➤ Strategic planning and organizational evaluation

In addition to *Innovative Staffing for the Medical Practice*, Dr. Keegan has co-authored four other best-selling MGMA books: *Rightsizing: Appropriate Staffing for Your Medical Practice, The Physician Billing*

Process: 12 Potholes to Avoid in the Road to Getting Paid (1st and 2nd editions), and *Physician Compensation Plans: State-of-the-Art Strategies.*

Dr. Keegan earned her PhD studying under Peter Drucker and other management scholars at the Peter F. Drucker Graduate School of Management. She received her MBA from UCLA's Anderson Graduate School of Management, and she is a Fellow of the American College of Medical Practice Executives.

With rich experience in consulting, education, and industry research, Dr. Keegan brings knowledge, expertise, and solutions to healthcare organizations. Her goal is to not only help organizations be relevant and successful today, but also to position organizations for the future as they work to meet the healthcare needs of their communities.

To contact Dr. Keegan or learn more about her services, go to www.deborahwalkerkeegan.com.

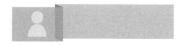

Table of Contents

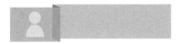

Introduction

Your staff are the infrastructure and support for physician productivity and practice efficiency. Importantly, they are also instrumental in providing quality and personalized care to your patients.

This book addresses two key questions as you staff your medical practice for optimal performance:

- ➤ Do you have the right staff?
- ➤ Are the staff doing the right things?

Both questions need to be asked and answered to create an innovative staffing model for your medical practice that is optimal for provider productivity and efficiency, practice profitability, staff recruitment and retention, and patient value.

The first question relates to the number of staff in the medical practice and the skill mix of these staff. In this book, we share two methods to approach this assessment. The first involves comparing your staff with benchmark data relating to the number of staff, the skill mix of staff, and the cost of staff in your medical practice. The second method involves analyzing the current workload of your staff and comparing it with expected staff workload ranges.

The second question, are the staff doing the right things, relates to the staffing deployment model you have implemented in your medical practice and the actual work that you have assigned to your staff. We share staffing deployment models and streamlined work processes so that you can determine whether your staffing organization and work assignments are optimal. We present innovative staffing strategies to help you imagine other ways to staff your medical practice to position it for future success. Innovative staffing strategies are provided to help you staff the telephones, the front office, the visit, the billing office, and medical records. Recognizing that today's medical practice needs to be flexible and agile, we present innovative staffing strategies for fluctuating work levels and the role of part-time and virtual staff, along with a discussion of the best ways to grow, hire, and share staff and outsource work functions.

Medical practices are increasingly embracing innovative staffing models and strategies. In some cases, they have redesigned the patient flow process and, consequently, the staff roles and work functions involved in patient flow. In other cases, they have altered their staffing strategy due to electronic health records. And in still other cases, staffing models have been changed to recognize changes in the healthcare reimbursement environment, such as consumer-driven health plans and pay-for-performance. Changes to staffing models to align the medical practice with these changes are presented throughout this book.

Although it is important to have the right staff and ensure they are doing the right thing, we also need to recognize that we need the very best and brightest staff in our medical practices today. We have devoted chapters to talent management and staff compensation and incentive plans. It is difficult to recruit staff who have the knowledge and expertise needed for today's medical practices. At the same time, it is incumbent on us to educate our staff so that they can be the very best they can be.

The book is organized into six parts:

Part 1: Staffing the Medical Practice. In Chapter 1, we present an overview of optimal staffing strategies and key areas of consideration as you staff your medical practice. In Chapter 2, we discuss changes in the healthcare delivery and reimbursement environments and the need to staff for these changes now — or risk becoming irrelevant. We proceed through the steps of analyzing a staffing deployment model for a medical practice in Chapter 3, where we array a staffing model and ask and answer critical questions to determine staffing improvement.

Part 2: Do You Have the Right Staff? The second part of the book is devoted to answering this question. In this section, we discuss two separate models for analyzing staff volume and skill mix. In Chapter 4, we present the staff benchmarking process and learn how to compare a medical practice's staffing with benchmark survey instruments. Recognizing the limitations to staff benchmarking, in Chapter 5, we build the required staffing model for the work that has been delegated to the staff. We present expected staff workload ranges for each of the key work functions in a medical practice and then build the staffing model that is needed for the work.

Part 3: Are the Staff Doing the Right Things? We address this question by presenting functional innovation, that is, innovative staffing strategies for key work functions in a medical practice. For each work function, we identify the unit of work, specific work tasks, and expected workload and performance measures. We then build a staff model based on the work and discuss staffing innovations that can better align your medical practice for future success. Chapters are devoted to each of the key work functions in a medical practice as follows: creating a care team (Chapter 6), staffing the telephones (Chapter 7), staffing the front office (Chapter 8), staffing the visit (Chapter 9), staffing the billing office (Chapter 10), staffing for medical records and electronic health records (Chapter 11), and staffing the medical home model (Chapter 12).

Part 4: Innovative Strategies to Optimize Flexibility and Leverage Physicians. Innovative staffing strategies to optimize flexibility and to leverage physicians are the work of the fourth section of the book. In this section on flexible innovation, we discuss staffing for fluctuating work levels (Chapter 13), the use of part-time and virtual staff (Chapter 14), and role options for nonphysician providers (Chapter 15).

A medical practice may need to revisit historical models in order to truly leverage the physician and assimilate the nonphysician provider as a member of the care team.

Part 5: Process Improvement. Many of the work processes we use in the medical practice are cumbersome and out of date. The actual work processes provided to the staff play a large role in the staffing model that is needed for a medical practice. Medical practices with encumbered processes typically require more staff than medical practices that have streamlined their work processes. Thus, the fifth section of the book is devoted to work process redesign, involving lean thinking and a systematic approach to creating intentional discipline in work (Chapter 16). We also discuss the need to connect staff to the purpose of a medical practice (Chapter 17) and remind staff each and every day of the good works they accomplish in service to their patients.

Part 6: Staff Recruitment, Recognition, and Retention. The final section of the book is devoted to staff recruitment, recognition, and retention. We discuss the merits and approaches to growing, hiring, and sharing staff, as well as outsourcing work in a medical practice. High performers are the focus of this section and the importance of dealing with Nurse Betty Behaving Badly is a central theme, as we discuss talent management and staff compensation and incentive plans to reward and recognize staff in the medical practice.

The following five themes are continuously addressed in this book:

Staff for the Work

The traditional staffing models that assign staff to specific physicians or tasks for each day of the week and each session per day are outdated. In today's medical practice, staff need to be flexibly deployed to manage the work on a given day or a given session per day.

This may include assigning more staff to work the telephones on Monday morning when typically the heaviest inbound telephone volume is received, rather than sustain the high level of staffing required for Monday mornings throughout the workweek. This also includes consolidating scheduling, referral management, telephone management, and other similar functions to permit economies of scale and scope, compared with a one-to-one assignment of a staff member to a physician or to a specific work function. In this fashion, the medical practice is staffed for the actual work that needs to be performed.

You Are Doing the Work Anyway

Throughout this book we recommend changes to a staff member's work scope and responsibilities. In many cases, this is to create a proactive, systematic approach to the work rather than fix errors on the back end or work in a frenetic fashion.

For example, we advocate conducting patient financial clearance prior to the patient being seen to ensure that a clean claim is submitted to the payer and that time-of-service payment obligations are met. If this work is not performed before the patient is seen, your medical practice will still be doing the work, as staff will need to be deployed in the billing office to work claim denials and to follow up with the patient to obtain payment. Thus, you are doing the work anyway. The determination of when the work is performed needs to be made. In this example, the decision is whether you want to pull the work into the medical practice and conduct it in a proactive, planned fashion or push the work to the back of the process and respond to claim denials from payers. Either way, the work is being done. But the success of the work efforts is higher and the cost to perform the work is lower in the former instance, where the work can be conducted in a proactive and planned approach.

Adopt a Patient Lens

In this book, we emphasize a patient-centric approach to patient flow. The patient is placed at the center of the patient flow process, with a physician-led care team working in coordination to provide value to the patient. This is at odds with a number of medical practices that place the physician or nurse at the center of the process. By placing the patient at the center of patient flow we can redesign our care processes and redeploy the staff to meet patient needs.

It Takes a Team

We emphasize the importance of teamwork in the medical practice. Given the choice among people, price, place, or product (or, in the case of medical practices, service), it is the people that make a difference in the medical practice. As one colleague recently remarked, "we may forget names and faces, but we always remember how people made us feel." In medical practices, it is important to remember our true purpose — to meet the healthcare needs of our communities. This requires a well-coordinated care team that is both professional and empathic. People are our core competency and it takes a team (and, consistent with the "it takes a village" analogy, increasingly, a medical home and a medical neighborhood) of dedicated professionals to make a difference in patients' lives.

Expect Staff Contribution

Expect more from your staff — they have significant strengths and the creativity, innovation, and intellectual capital to help you build a great medical practice. Don't just tap into it; embrace employees as partners in your medical practice, focus on selective recruitment, and expect high levels of engagement and contribution.

With these themes prominent in this book, we present tools and techniques to innovate and optimize the staffing strategy for your medical practice.

PART 1

Staffing the Medical Practice

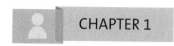

CHAPTER 1

Optimal Staffing for the Medical Practice: An Overview

What is our goal? The right number of staff, in the right place, with the right skills, at the right cost, with the right behavior, with the right rewards, with the right outcomes. No more, no less.

—Rightsizing: Appropriate Staffing for Your Medical Practice

We have had the opportunity to observe a number of missteps medical practices have taken as they work to staff the medical practice, as well as a number of stellar organizations that have managed to get it right. Due to the changes in healthcare today, we are witnessing a revolution in staffing for the medical practice. There are new patient access channels, new patient flow processes, and new knowledge and skill needs — all of which impact the staffing deployment model and the staffing strategy you adopt for your medical practice.

In this chapter, we discuss:

- ➤ The importance of appropriate staffing
- ➤ The consequences of inappropriate staffing levels

➤ The consequences of inappropriate skill mix

➤ Staffing for three patient flow processes: internal, external, and virtual patient flows

IMPORTANCE OF APPROPRIATE STAFFING

Why should we be concerned about correctly staffing the medical practice? After all, shouldn't each medical practice determine this for itself? The staffing roles and responsibilities and staffing deployment models vary from one practice to the next, but the important point is to ensure that your medical practice has evaluated its infrastructure and support to the billable provider and that you have assessed and concluded that your practice, indeed, has the right staff doing the right things.

Staff are instrumental in ensuring quality clinical care and they are the conduit by which patients access their care. They also manage the business of medicine functions, so that today's medical practices can remain in business to see patients. If we staff the medical practice correctly, these staff can work in a coordinated and cohesive fashion to ensure that provider and patient needs are met, thereby streamlining the patient flow process. Correctly staffing the medical practice results in optimized patient care and service.

Data suggest that appropriate staffing for a medical practice permits physicians (or other providers) to optimize their productivity and efficiency. This is not trivial. The chief constraint in a medical practice is the physician's time. Once a schedule is not full or a patient fails to keep his or her appointment, that time is gone — it cannot be inventoried.[1] Though some staff are deployed in support of the physician and enable the physician to provide clinical services, the vast majority of functions carried out by the staff in a medical practice are administrative. Indeed, the only truly value-added steps in the

---

[1] A detailed discussion of this concept can be found in Woodcock, Elizabeth W. 2009. *Mastering Patient Flow: Using Lean Thinking to Improve Your Practice Operations, 3rd Edition.* Englewood, Colo.: Medical Group Management Association.

entire patient flow process from the patient's point of view is the actual time the patient spends in the exam room with the physician or when receiving care via virtual medicine (for example, receiving clinical information and instruction via a telephone visit, secure message, or patient Web portal).

Medical practices that are appropriately staffed recognize the following two key advantages:

> *Physician time is optimized.* There is less wasted time and tasks are delegated to the appropriate level based on licensure and type of work.

> *Physicians are able to focus on clinical care.* Physicians are able to effectively use their distinct competencies to evaluate, diagnose, and treat patients.

> Indeed, the only truly value-added steps in the entire patient flow process from the patient's point of view is the actual time the patient spends in the exam room with the physician or when receiving care via virtual medicine.

CONSEQUENCES OF INAPPROPRIATE STAFFING LEVELS

There are a number of negative consequences if your medical practice has either too few staff or too many staff members.

An insufficient volume of staff to carry out the work may result in the following negative consequences for a medical practice:

> *Staff recruitment and retention problems.* Prospective employees are not keen to work in a medical practice where staff are overextended and overstressed. Similarly, current employees — often your best and brightest — can recognize that there are jobs outside your practice where their talent and expertise can be used in more meaningful ways.

➤ *Poor patient service.* It is just not possible for each and every staff member who is overextended to provide a consistent level of service and support to the patient, let alone the physician. As a consequence, customer service declines and can deteriorate to levels where patients no longer want to be seen by your physicians. Service is often considered a proxy for quality. Thus, if service is suboptimal, patients will often interpret this to mean that quality, too, is below par.

➤ *Increased business risk.* We often see staff performing "out of class" in medical practices with too few staff. That is, a medical assistant starts to resemble a licensed nurse by inappropriately providing clinical advice to the patient. Or, a nurse practitioner may perform simple nursing tasks, such as telephone triage or even room a patient, which also is another form of out-of-class work. We often also witness work falling through the cracks. Staff just don't have time to address certain key functions, such as following up with a no-show patient to determine why he or she missed the appointment and rescheduling that patient for needed care, or tracking down a missing test result. Business risk increases and quality and safety can be compromised by staffing at an inappropriately low level.

➤ *High levels of multitasking.* A fourth consequence of too few staff is that staff members are basically assigned to do everything, with the expectation that they will get to it when they can. This results in loss of accountability and work discipline. Some work does not get done and, when it is performed, it may be of inconsistent quality.

➤ *Inefficient physicians.* Lastly, in medical practices with too few staff, we often witness a physician performing nonclinical, administrative tasks. Work that could be delegated is not delegated; there is no one who can take on the task. We witness a domino effect: declining physician productivity negatively impacts patient access and, in turn, negatively impacts the financial viability of the practice. There is slow exam-room turnover and limited visit assistance when there are too few staff to manage the work inherent in ambulatory care.

We often see the ratio of new patients to return patients decline, and there is a tendency to inappropriately close the practice to new patients, simply because there is insufficient infrastructure. True, we want a lean staff, but we need the staff to be optimally effective.

> Service is often considered a proxy for quality. Thus, if service is sub-optimal, patients will often interpret this to mean that quality, too, is below par.

Too many staff at work in a medical practice also can lead to negative consequences, including:

➤ *High staff cost.* When there are too many staff, there is commonly low staff productivity, yet staffing costs (and therefore overhead costs) are higher than peer practices, negatively impacting the profitability of the medical practice and thereby impacting the ability to effectively compete for patients or hire new physicians. In these medical practices, the cost of staff as a percentage of total medical revenue is higher than benchmark norms. The cost of staff for most medical practices is 30 percent or more of total medical revenue generated by the medical practice. This is an expense only exceeded by provider cost.[2] Staff are a major investment, and it is important for a medical practice to staff correctly to identify the right staff and have them doing the right things in order to optimize practice efficiency and profitability and to ensure patients receive quality care and service.

➤ *Inability to ratchet up productivity.* A second consequence of too many staff is the missing link between staff and the work. The

---

[2] Benchmark data reflecting the cost of support staff as a percentage of total medical revenue are available in the following MGMA survey instruments published annually: *Cost Survey for Multispecialty Practices, Cost Survey for Single-Specialty Practices,* and *Performance and Practices of Successful Medical Groups.* In addition, MGMA publishes specialty-specific surveys in key specialties. See the Additional Resources list at the end of this book for details regarding these survey instruments.

low levels of staff productivity get ingrained into the mind-set of staff, and any effort to increase productivity is met with resistance and entrenchment. The staff have gotten used to a certain pace and method of doing things that cannot be real-istically sustained, and staff productivity per unit of work de-clines. One of the toughest challenges for any medical practice is to ratchet up productivity once staff are used to working at a certain pace.

➤ *Increase in human resources challenges.* In medical practices with too many staff, it seems that the staff have too much time on their hands. They create human resources challenges at a level not found in many other medical practices that have managed to staff correctly.

➤ *Moral hazard.* In medical practices with high staff volumes, we often see shirking behavior from some staff who do not pull their weight and participate as equal members of the care team. This can have a negative impact on team behavior and the ability to retain high-performing team members.

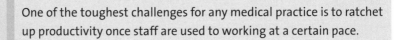

One of the toughest challenges for any medical practice is to ratchet up productivity once staff are used to working at a certain pace.

CONSEQUENCES OF INAPPROPRIATE SKILL MIX

There are also consequences to a medical practice when an incor-rect skill mix or licensure of staff is deployed. Many of the negative consequences that result when medical practices have too few or too many staff members also apply when there is an improper skill mix of staff. For example, staff may perform out of class. This is a costly staffing model in which licensed staff perform routine tasks that can be delegated to other, less-qualified staff or, alternatively, when staff are asked to perform work that is beyond their level of competency. This can lead to business risk in a medical practice, a high-cost staffing model, and inappropriate support for the provider. It can also negatively impact patient safety and quality service.

As this discussion demonstrates, the staff in a medical practice play a vital role in its success. The impact of incorrect staffing is detrimental to the medical practice, negatively impacting staff recruitment and retention, medical practice productivity and profitability, patient care and safety, and patient perceptions of service. The consequences of inappropriate staffing of a medical practice are summarized in Exhibit 1.1.

EXHIBIT 1.1	Consequences of Inappropriate Staffing
Too few staff	→ Low physician productivity → Problem recruitment and retention → Poor patient care and service → Increased business risk
Too many staff	→ Low staff productivity → High cost → Inappropriate work scope → More human resources challenges → Moral hazard
Inappropriate skill mix of staff	→ Increased business risk → High cost → Inappropriate work scope → Low physician productivity → Poor patient care and service

Adapted with permission from Walker, Deborah L., and David N. Gans. 2003. *Rightsizing: Appropriate Staffing for Your Medical Practice*. Englewood, Colo.: Medical Group Management Association.

STAFFING FOR THREE PATIENT FLOW PROCESSES

In today's medical practices, we need to deploy the staff and harness their talents and contributions to optimally support three patient flow processes: (1) the internal patient flow process, (2) the external patient flow process, and (3) the virtual patient flow process (see Exhibit 1.2).

> → *The internal patient flow process.* The internal patient flow process involves the work that occurs during a face-to-face visit with a patient, including patient check-in, patient retrieval, rooming and work-up, the visit itself, and patient check-out.

> → *The external patient flow process.* The external patient flow process primarily involves the management of inbound telephone calls from patients, including telephone scheduling, telephone messaging, and telephone nurse triage. The external patient flow process also includes non–face-to-face business transactions with the patient through written or oral communication such as referral and authorization management and billing and collection functions.

> → *The virtual patient flow process.* In today's delivery system, there is a third patient flow process: the virtual patient flow process. The Web portal, virtual visits with physicians, care and case management, health coaching and outreach, and secure message threads with the care team require a distinct focus of staff roles and responsibilities. Whether using a Web portal, smart phone, or social media such as blogs and tweets, these methods of communication and access need to be supported by qualified staff.

> In addition to staffing the face-to-face visit and the telephones, we need to staff for virtual medicine. The Web portal, virtual visits with providers, care and case management, health coaching and outreach, and secure message threads with the care team require a distinct focus of staff roles and responsibilities.

Each of these patient flow processes — internal, external, and virtual — must be aligned and optimally staffed in order to streamline the patient flow process and optimize patient value. We need the right staff doing the right things so that we can provide the right care at the right cost for our patients.

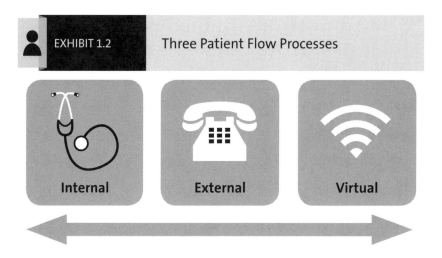

EXHIBIT 1.2   Three Patient Flow Processes

Internal   External   Virtual

SUMMARY

As we have discussed in this chapter, it is important for a medical practice to staff correctly — to assemble the appropriate volume of staff with the right skill mix. There are negative consequences for having too many or too few staff, not the least of which are problematic physician productivity and efficiency and negative impacts to quality care and patient service. In today's medical practice, support staff need to be optimally deployed to manage three distinct patent flow processes — internal, external, and virtual patient flows — to ensure that the medical practice is relevant and aligned with changes in the healthcare delivery system.

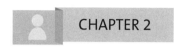

CHAPTER 2

Staffing for the Future Now

The important thing is to identify the future that has already happened.

—Peter F. Drucker

Medical practices have traditionally provided services to their patients via face-to-face visits scheduled on an episodic basis. Today, an expanded array of patient access options is available, and new staffing models are needed to manage the changes in the delivery system and the changes in healthcare financing and reimbursement models.

In this chapter, we discuss the need to change staff roles and responsibilities for the following six specific changes occurring in today's healthcare environment:

- ➤ Virtual medicine

- ➤ Patient-centered medical homes

- ➤ Expanded patient access channels

- ➤ Consumer-directed health plans

- ➤ Pay-for-value reimbursement

- ➤ Accountable care

STAFFING STRATEGIES FOR VIRTUAL MEDICINE

Many medical practices now offer patients virtual medicine. This includes:

- Secure message threads sent between the patient and the care team
- 24/7 nurse and physician management of the patient via telephone
- Outreach care management and health and wellness coaching
- Telemedicine involving portable mobile devices (mobile health), video, and other technologies

Staff need to be deployed to schedule the telephone visit, respond to inbound telephone calls, respond to secure message threads, set up video conferencing, and other similar work in order to facilitate virtual medicine. The work involved in supporting virtual medicine cannot simply be piled higher and higher on the staff involved in the face-to-face patient visit. Instead, a formal staffing plan and staffing deployment model are required. This involves a redistribution of work tasks, roles, and responsibilities in order to effectively staff for this work. We discuss staffing for virtual medicine in Chapter 11, Staffing for Medical Records and Electronic Health Records, and in Chapter 12, Staffing the Medical Home Model.

STAFFING STRATEGIES FOR THE PATIENT-CENTERED MEDICAL HOME

Many medical practices are piloting patient-centered medical home models. In these models, a care team works to ensure that patients are highly engaged and active in their care. Patients have access to care 24/7 and a team of physicians and staff, to include care and case managers, health and wellness coaches, psychologists, pharmacists, social workers, and telephone nurse triage staff are assembled to work with patients to help them maintain their health and wellness and manage transitions of care. In turn, there are expectations for the patients to use expanded access methods to interact with their care team beyond the face-to-face, episodic visit of the traditional medical practice and become active in self-care.

Staffing strategies in medical home models are different from the traditional staffing model of a medical practice in the following ways:

> ➤ Nursing staff are assigned to manage inbound calls and secure message threads using a "real-time, one-touch" strategy

> ➤ Medical assistants prepare for the visit by accessing registries and care tools to determine outstanding services required for the patient

> ➤ The status of the patient is routinely reviewed by the care team, with next steps actively managed and communicated to the patient

> ➤ Transitions of care from primary care to specialty care to hospital care to nursing home to home health are coordinated by staff assigned to this function

In short, rather than having patients "go fish" for information or manage their own transitions of care, a care team is deployed to assist patients throughout their journey to health and wellness. In Chapter 12, we detail staffing strategies for the medical home model.

STAFFING STRATEGIES FOR EXPANDED PATIENT ACCESS

Today's medical practices are expanding patient access channels to ensure that patients are engaged and active in their care. Staffing deployment models in the medical practice must change to meet the needs of patients and manage these access methods. For example, staff need to be assigned to manage the following:

> ➤ The medical practice's Web portal

> ➤ Secure online messaging systems

> ➤ Telephone visits and e-visits

> ➤ Telephone nursing and care management

➤ Self-directed care

➤ Individualized, patient-specific care

These work functions are in addition to the staff needed to provide the infrastructure and support for the face-to-face patient visit.

Today's medical practices are expanding patient access channels to ensure that patients are engaged and active in their care.

Support staff in today's medical practices must be able to work in a well-coordinated team to manage this expanded patient access model of care. Exhibit 2.1 describes the various delivery system models of today's medical practices.

We review innovative staffing strategies to manage these and other expanded patient access channels in the pertinent chapters of this book. It is important to note here, however, that staffing models must change in a medical practice in response to these changes in patient access modalities, which have been designed to better meet patient needs for quality, low-cost care. This involves changing the staffing deployment model and work assignment of staff to manage new roles and responsibilities in the medical practice.

STAFFING STRATEGIES FOR CONSUMER-DIRECTED HEALTH PLANS

Patients are paying more and more out of pocket for their care. In addition to higher premiums, consumer-directed healthcare plans require patients to personally select a mix of premium, deductible, co-insurance, and copayment. Many of these plans involve a high deductible, which must be met by the patient prior to any insurance payment for the service.

What this means for the medical practice is that patients are more financially engaged in their care and more of the medical practice's revenue is derived from patients. Although the patient may have

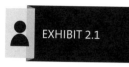

Delivery System	Functions
Web portal	E-consults E-visits Patient health record, logs, journals Patient portal Secure messaging Online appointment scheduling Online test results reporting Online prescription management Online education
Telephone visits, mobile health	Virtual visits with provider Nurse advice and consultation Care management
Video visits	Remote access Telemedicine
Self-directed care	Online wellness plans Telediagnostics management Device and skin patch management Self-testing and self-management
Patient outreach	Patient recall Expanded referral methods Health and wellness coaching

private insurance, if he or she has a $5,000 deductible plan, the vast majority of healthcare in a given year may in actuality be "self-pay" or the patient's out-of-pocket responsibility. This is challenging for medical practices that typically have tight margins and must now attempt to collect more than a copayment from patients at the point of care (provided third-party payer contracts permit this to occur). Collecting from patients after services are performed is more difficult and costly than collecting from patients when they are in the medical practice. Consequently, changes to the staffing model and the work processes assigned to the staff are required in order to understand the patient's insurance and point-of-care payment obligations.

We recommend that staff be assigned to conduct the work of patient financial clearance prior to the patient being seen. This includes insurance verification, benefits eligibility, prior account balance identification, and other similar work. If the decision is made not to conduct patient financial clearance, the work is still being performed, it is just a different kind of work at a higher cost. In this example, if patient financial clearance is not performed to ensure that a clean claim is submitted to the payer, billing staff need to be deployed to appeal a claim that may have been denied due to incorrect insurance, coverage requirements, patient deductible, or other reasons.

This discussion is consistent with one of the themes of this book: "you are doing the work anyway." It is simply a different timing and approach to the work and, consequently, a different staffing deployment model to ensure the work is done earlier in the process (prior to the elective service being performed), rather than later (after the claim has been submitted, adjudicated, and denied).

Examples of the work required for patient financial clearance in markets where consumer-directed healthcare is prevalent are listed in Exhibit 2.2. The work of patient financial clearance is typically managed by front office staff; however, some medical practices will involve billing office staff, as well. The various staffing strategies in use today to conduct patient financial clearance functions are described in Chapter 8, Staffing the Front Office.

Beyond patient financial clearance and the changing role of staff to manage this process, we are beginning to see payers experiment with real-time claims adjudication. In real-time claims adjudication, a large portion of the billing is conducted at patient check-out, where the claim information is entered into the payer Website, with immediate notification to the medical practice of the amount to

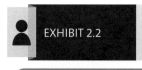

EXHIBIT 2.2

Patient Financial Clearance Work Functions

Patient Financial Clearance

- Insurance verification
- Benefits eligibility
  - Authorization
  - Waivers
- Financial responsibility
  - Account balance
  - Copayment level
  - Co-insurance, deductible
  - Credit worthiness
  - Financial risk assessment
- Patient no-show history

collect from the patient at the point of care (and the balance of the allowable transferred by the payer to your medical practice's bank account). This is another example of our theme of "you are doing the work anyway." Instead of staffing the billing office to perform a significant portion of these functions, the work is performed at the practice site, and billing is conducted in real time in the physical presence of the patient. If this model becomes prominent, it will truly revolutionize staffing of the revenue cycle in today's medical practices. See Chapter 10, Staffing the Billing Office, for more staffing innovations for the physician billing process.

STAFFING STRATEGIES FOR PAY-FOR-VALUE REIMBURSEMENT

Healthcare reimbursement models are also changing. As more and more payers elect to pay differentially based on performance or value (typically referred to as pay-for-performance or pay-for-value plans), the work of staff in the medical practice needs to be altered to ensure that physicians and the medical practice can demonstrate performance and outcomes consistent with quality and cost targets and/or demonstrate performance that is of high value (particularly if plans are constructed to share cost savings).

To be successful in a pay-for-value environment with "at-risk" reimbursement, the following three changes to staffing deployment models are required:

- Staff involved in evidence-based patient care and patient activation
- Staff involved in program development and infrastructure
- Coding staff (for procedure coding as well as diagnosis coding, which begins the algorithm for differential reimbursement)

Each of these changes to staffing deployment models is discussed in the following sections.

Evidence-Based Patient Care and Patient Activation

The work of ensuring that the patient's care and treatment are consistent with evidence-based guidelines and established targets and goals rests with the physician and clinical support staff, necessitating a change to staffing work scope and effort. A pay-for-value plan requires that clinical protocols and evidence-based guidelines be followed and that documentation be secured to demonstrate patient outcomes. Electronic health records can assist in identifying outstanding clinical services required of patients, and disease and care registries and patient recall methods can also be used to support this work.

In medical practices without electronic tools, staff use clinical flow sheets designed for each patient to proactively oversee and manage care to ensure that the interventions occur and outcomes are reported, with data often entered into a patient registry or spreadsheet.

Clinical support staff in a medical practice play a major role in preparing for the visit and ensuring that the clinical protocols are followed and that the documentation is provided to demonstrate patient compliance, intervention, and outcomes. The role of the clinical support staff thus has increased in medical practices with pay-for-value plans. They must become highly involved in visit preparation, patient outreach, patient education, and patient self-management.

> The work of ensuring that the patient's care and treatment are consistent with evidence-based guidelines and established targets and goals rests with the provider and clinical support staff, necessitating a change to staffing work scope and effort.

Examples of work functions and tasks that are needed to demonstrate appropriate clinical intervention and outcomes are shown in Exhibit 2.3.

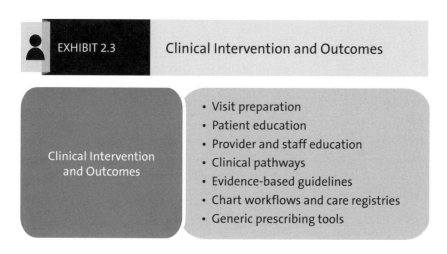

EXHIBIT 2.3   Clinical Intervention and Outcomes

Clinical Intervention and Outcomes

- Visit preparation
- Patient education
- Provider and staff education
- Clinical pathways
- Evidence-based guidelines
- Chart workflows and care registries
- Generic prescribing tools

See Chapter 9, Staffing the Visit, for a discussion of new roles of clinical support staff related to pay-for-value and other similar at-risk reimbursement models.

Infrastructure and Program Development

Program infrastructure for pay-for-value schemes also changes the staffing pattern in a medical practice in the following ways:

- ➤ In some cases, the number of information technology staff increases or the staff become more sophisticated due to the need to track and document the use of generic drugs, patient-specific interventions, and other data.

- ➤ In other cases, nurse coordinators are hired to manage the pay-for-value program. This involves determining complete-ness of care pursuant to established clinical protocols, en-gaging physicians in care delivery, monitoring quality outcomes and measures, and other important roles as part of the contractual obligation for the pay-for-value plan with the payer.

- ➤ Pay-for-value program staff are also typically hired to deter-mine performance targets and metrics, create operational definitions of the metrics, and educate physicians regarding the measures.

- ➤ Staff are also required for data analysis and management reporting. Physicians need to routinely receive their perfor-mance outcomes to learn their progress toward established targets and goals and to permit course corrections.

In short, medical practices that participate in risk-based reimburse-ment need to assign staff to support the patient visit and the medi-cal practice in new ways in order to help the physicians and achieve financial success.

Coding Support

Another changing role that is often overlooked by medical practices as they successfully contract for pay-for-value plans is that of cod-ing support. Typically, the diagnosis code, which in many medical practices is determined by physicians (and increasingly and inappropriately by clinical support staff, reception staff, and a host of others who are not trained in this determination), becomes an important element in the algorithm used to determine pay-for-value reimbursement. Consequently, pay-for-value plans often require dedicated certified coders to ensure that the work performed by the physicians is accurately reflected through both diagnosis and procedure codes. This work is likely to be heightened with the implementation of International Classification of Diseases, Tenth Revision (ICD-10) diagnostic coding and the resulting demands for a higher level of code specificity than required by the current ICD-9 classification system.

> Medical practices that participate in risk-based reimbursement need to assign staff to support the patient visit and the medical practice in new ways in order to support the physicians and achieve financial success.

STAFFING STRATEGIES TO DEMONSTRATE ACCOUNTABLE CARE

Is your medical practice providing "accountable care"?[1] That is, can you truly demonstrate the quality and cost of the care that you provide to ensure that you are indeed providing value to patients? In today's medical practices, online registries and other electronic tools have become prominent in ensuring that medical practices demonstrate value and deliver quality and coordinated care. Managing and maintaining data and extracting and reporting information from patient care records are now expected components of the way we do business in today's medical practice.

---

[1] The term *accountable care* is typically used to describe a reimbursement methodology for organizations that have assumed responsibility for a patient population. In this chapter, the term is used to draw attention to the fact that, increasingly, medical practices need to demonstrate patient value (defined as high quality at low cost).

There are a number of federal demonstration projects underway to determine a different method of reimbursing medical practices beyond the currently prominent fee-for-service method. These include (1) shared incentives between hospitals and physicians, (2) a prospective, bundled payment for an acute episode of care involving hospital and physician services, and (3) fee-for-service plus arrangements involving a care or case management fee. Staffing to ensure that the medical practice performs the appropriate work and, importantly, achieves the expected clinical and patient outcomes of that work will require new staffing models and a redelegation of staff roles and responsibilities.

Beyond changes to the work of clinical support staff, this requires deployment of staff in clinical information systems, data and decision support and analysis, and similar venues. This also requires that the data be translated to usable information so that others can easily understand the cost, quality, productivity, and safety of delivered care. New roles and responsibilities for information technology and data support staff are inherent in accountable models of care.

SUMMARY

As we discussed in this chapter, changing delivery systems and changing reimbursement models have a direct impact on the staffing deployment model of a medical practice and the work functions and tasks delegated to staff. Today's medical practices must deploy appropriate staff resources to new work functions to ensure that the practice is aligned with the changes in the healthcare environment. In the following chapters, we explore innovative staffing strategies for key work functions in the medical practice.

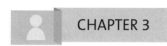

CHAPTER 3

How to Analyze Your Staffing Deployment Model

The first question to ask is "why"? Why have you adopted this particular staffing deployment model for your medical practice?

—Deborah Walker Keegan, PhD, FACMPE

A staffing deployment model outlines the staffing levels and work assignments a medical practice has adopted for key work functions. It identifies the "who" and the "how" work is to be performed.

In this chapter, we:

- ➤ Define staffing deployment models
- ➤ Learn how to analyze a staffing deployment model
- ➤ Describe the drawbacks to a traditional staffing deployment model
- ➤ Describe the steps needed to optimize staffing in the medical practice

STAFFING DEPLOYMENT MODELS

A staffing deployment model is the model that describes your staff and their assigned roles and responsibilities. Rarely will two medical practices have the exact same staffing model. The examples in

Exhibits 3.1 and 3.2 demonstrate the variation in staffing deployment models. Exhibit 3.1 reflects two separate staffing deployment models for front office work, and Exhibit 3.2 reflects two models for clinical support.

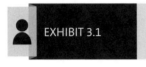

EXHIBIT 3.1   Front Office Staffing Model

Medical Practice A. In this medical practice, front office staff have been tasked with managing inbound telephone calls and conducting patient check-in.

Medical Practice B. In this medical practice, one set of staff is assigned to manage the inbound telephone calls and a second set of staff is assigned to conduct patient check-in. The roles do not overlap.

EXHIBIT 3.2   Clinical Support Staffing Model

Medical Practice A. In this medical practice, a nurse is assigned to work with one physician. The nurse performs an expanded work scope that includes rooming the patient, supporting the physician and the visit, and managing inbound telephone calls of a clinical nature.

Medical Practice B. In this medical practice, one nurse is assigned to manage the inbound telephone calls for four physicians. A medical assistant is assigned to retrieve and room the patient. The medical assistants work in pods (for example, one of three medical assistants may assist with patient rooming for a single physician).

As demonstrated by these examples, each of these medical practices has a different staffing deployment model and a different definition of who is involved in the work function and how that work function is to be carried out.

> A staffing deployment model is the model that describes your staff and their assigned roles and responsibilities.

ANALYZING YOUR STAFFING DEPLOYMENT MODEL

There are two basic steps to analyze your staffing deployment model. The first step is to array your current model. The second step is to ask and answer a specific set of questions in order to understand your current model and assess the changes that can be made to improve your model for the future. Each step is described below.

Step 1: Array Your Current Staffing Deployment Model

The first step in analyzing a medical practice's staffing deployment model is to array the model in a grid. A sample staffing deployment model is arrayed in Exhibit 3.3. The first column describes the work function. The second column describes who is performing each function. The last column is a summary of how that work function is currently performed.

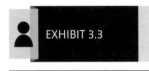

EXHIBIT 3.3   Staffing Deployment Model

Work Function	Who	How
Telephones	Front desk staff manage inbound telephone calls	The telephones ring in the reception area and are managed by the check-in/check-out staff
Patient check-in	Front desk staff manage patient check-in	Check-in staff verify and update information with the patient, conduct insurance verification, and obtain time-of-service payments
Patient check-out	Front desk staff manage patient check-out	Check-out staff schedule follow-up visits, manage outbound referrals, and conduct charge entry
Clinical support	There is a 1-to-1 assignment of a nurse to a physician	The nurse is responsible for both telephone calls and patient visit support

This staffing deployment model provides significant information about the medical practice. This medical practice has combined the staffing roles for both the internal and external patient flow processes as follows:

> ➤ Front office staff multitask to manage telephones and reception functions
> ➤ Clinical staff multitask to manage patient flow for the face-to-face visit in addition to telephone triage and advice support
> ➤ There are no virtual medicine or virtual patient flow processes

Step 2: Ask and Answer Questions Regarding Your Staffing Deployment Model

Once you have arrayed your staffing deployment model, the first question to ask and answer is, "why?" Why have you modeled your staff in this particular fashion? Often, the answer is that the staffing model was never proactively designed in the first place. Instead, over time, the medical practice grew, expanded, or changed, while the staffing model remained unchanged and now is no longer current.

By asking and answering a standard set of questions and comparing your staffing deployment model with those of other medical practices, you can determine if there are changes that can be made to your model that will be more effective in supporting the physician and the patient and better align your practice for the future.

> Over time, the medical practice grew, expanded, or changed, while the staffing model remained unchanged and now is no longer current.

Ask and answer the following questions as you analyze your staffing deployment model:

- *Work quantity.* Is the quantity of work consistent with the staff volume? (We discuss this concept further in Chapter 5, The Staff Workload Evaluation Process.)

- *Staff efficiency.* Are the staff efficient in the performance of their functions and tasks? Is there downtime? Are staff rushing around throughout the day or is there a systematic, planned, and focused approach to the work?

- *Work quality.* What is the work quality or outcome of the work? For example, what type of claim edits need to be worked due to problematic registration information? How many rings until the telephone is answered? What is the call abandonment rate? What is the lag time to return calls to patients? Is there a better way to staff the work function so that the work quality and quantity are consistent with expected levels?

➤ *Work backlog.* Is there work that is not being attended to on a regular basis? Are there work backlogs in key functional areas, such as scanning or patient recall?

➤ *Provider support.* Is the physician or nonphysician provider fully supported in the scope of his or her work? Is the provider wasting time looking for the nurse or obtaining his or her own patients, supplies, and materials for the visit?

➤ *Skill mix.* Are the nurses working in the full scope of licensure? Are they largely devoted to nursing tasks or to administrative tasks such as scheduling? Is a different skill set required for the work?

➤ *Work delegation.* What duties have providers delegated to staff? Are there additional duties that can be delegated to improve provider efficiency and patient access? Have the appropriate functions been delegated to the right level of staff in the medical practice?

➤ *Centralization and decentralization.* To what extent have specific work functions been centralized or decentralized? Would a change in centralization or decentralization enhance practice efficiency?

➤ *Care team.* Are the staff contributing to an integrated care team or are they functioning in silos? Can staff be co-located or can collaborative approaches to work be developed?

➤ *Economies of scale.* Is the practice taking advantage of economies of scale? Can work functions be linked with other staff or other parts of the medical practice?

➤ *Patient delegation.* Can patients perform some tasks themselves, for example, register via kiosk at the practice site, schedule appointments online, obtain test results online, update registration online, and room themselves?

➤ *Virtual medicine.* Can more virtual medicine be performed, such as secure messaging, telephone visits, proactive patient outreach, and health and wellness coaching?

By arraying your staffing deployment model and asking key questions, you begin to understand potential opportunities to improve the infrastructure and support for the physician and patient. You see the potential to change patient access channels and your care delivery system.

DRAWBACKS OF TRADITIONAL STAFFING DEPLOYMENT MODELS

In this chapter, we purposefully arrayed a traditional staffing deployment model. We devote the rest of this book to discussing more advanced and innovative staffing models that are better aligned with the changes in today's healthcare environment and that have proven to be successful in enhancing productivity, efficiency, patient access, and service.

The traditional staffing deployment model that was depicted in this chapter does not identify separate and distinct staff involved in the internal patient flow process (the visit) from that of the external patient flow process (the telephones). When a medical practice has this type of staffing deployment model, we typically observe less practice productivity and efficiency than in a medical practice with a more advanced staffing model. In medical practices with this traditional model, we typically observe the following:

➤ *High multitasking.* The front office staff are unable to be successful while simultaneously attending to telephones and the patients arriving for visits.

➤ *High claim edits and denials.* There are high claim edit and claim denial rates because the multitasking staff make more mistakes in collecting patients' demographic and insurance information.

➤ *Reduced time-of-service collections.* The amount of money collected at the point of care is lower than expected, due to the hectic pace of the front office and lack of business planning prior to patient visits.

➤ *Poor patient service.* The staff are rushed in their telephone interaction with patients, resulting in poor perceptions of service by patients. In addition, patients perceive a frenetic pace in the practice when they present for care.

➤ *Inefficient scheduling.* The staff are not able to optimize the scheduling template due to the competing demands for their time, resulting in physician inefficiency.

➤ *Failure to clinically prepare for the visit.* There is no clinical visit preparation because clinical support staff are required to manage both the telephones and patient flow for the visit and do not have the time to conduct this work.

➤ *Inefficient physicians.* The physician must wait for the patient to be checked in and roomed because of staffing inefficiencies at both the front desk and among clinical support staff.

➤ *Physicians leave exam rooms before exams are completed.* Physicians leave the exam room to "find nurse Betty," because the nurse is busy with telephone calls and piles of charts (or electronic in-box messages) and is not able to anticipate patient and physician needs for the visit.

> By arraying your staffing deployment model and asking key questions, you begin to understand potential opportunities to improve the infrastructure and support for the physician and patient.

Arraying your staffing deployment model and asking critical questions regarding each aspect of your model are the first actions to take to determine if you have optimized the staffing model in your medical practice. Exhibit 3.4 outlines the next four steps that need to be taken to fully analyze staffing opportunities and optimize your staffing model. The steps include:

1. *Benchmark staff full-time equivalents (FTEs) and costs.* Perform a gap analysis, comparing your staffing model with the benchmarks.

2. *Evaluate staff workload.* Compare the work quantity of your staff with expected staff workload ranges. Perform a gap analysis, comparing your staffing model with the expected workload ranges.

3. *Redesign work processes.* Identify opportunities to streamline work processes, reduce waste, and standardize the work performed by your staff.

4. *Innovate your model.* Use the staffing data and work process redesign to innovate the staffing model for your medical practice.

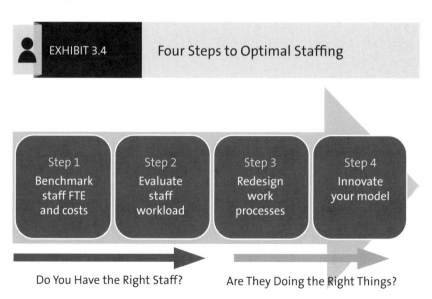

EXHIBIT 3.4   Four Steps to Optimal Staffing

| Step 1 Benchmark staff FTE and costs | Step 2 Evaluate staff workload | Step 3 Redesign work processes | Step 4 Innovate your model |

Do You Have the Right Staff?   Are They Doing the Right Things?

The first two steps help you answer the question "do I have the right staff in my practice?" Steps 3 and 4 help you answer the question "are the staff doing the right things?"

SUMMARY

In this chapter, we discussed the importance of arraying your current staffing deployment model and asking and answering important questions to help you determine improvements to your model. We also identified the drawbacks to a traditional staffing model. In the chapters that follow, we work through the four steps to optimal staffing to determine whether you have the right staff doing the right things in your practice.

PART 2

Do You Have the Right Staff?

Analyze Staff Volume and Skill Mix

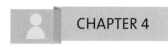

CHAPTER 4

The Staff Benchmarking Process

What you cannot measure you cannot manage.

—David N. Gans, MHSA, FACMPE
Vice President, Innovation and Research
Medical Group Management Association

There are two tools to address the question, "Do I have the right staff in my medical practice?" One tool is to benchmark your current staff with peer medical practices. The second tool is to compare the work-load of your staff to expected staff workload ranges. By utilizing both tools, a medical practice is able to target areas for potential staffing opportunity.

In this chapter, we present:

➢ What the benchmarks tell us

➢ Staff benchmark data

➢ Benchmark limitations

➢ Basic approach to staff benchmarking

WHAT THE BENCHMARKS TELL US

Benchmark staffing data help us to identify areas of opportunity for improving the staffing strategy in a medical practice. The benchmark data are available at the specialty level for most medical and surgical disciplines. From these data, we have learned a number of important lessons regarding staffing the medical practice for optimal performance.

Lesson 1: Specialty Distinctions

Medical practices staff at very different levels depending on their specialty. For example, a family medicine practice typically has more staff than a surgical practice such as urology. This is due to the fact that the family medicine physicians devote the majority of their time in the ambulatory care setting, whereas surgeons split their time between the clinic and the hospital, where they have a separate team to support their procedural and inpatient work.

Lesson 2: Variation Within the Same Specialties

Medical practices also staff at very different levels within the same specialty. We typically see a bell-shaped curve when we graph the staffing levels of all practices in a particular specialty. Exhibit 4.1 reflects this type of bell-shaped curve. Though the numbers and percentages reported in the graph change by specialty and over time, the graph generally maintains a bell shape regardless of specialty.

Lesson 3: Staffing at the Median

Many medical practices make the incorrect assumption that they should simply staff at benchmark median levels. This is the midpoint of the bell-shaped curve where one half of the practices in the dataset report fewer staff and one half of the practices report more staff than this midpoint level.

When medical practices revert to the median, they ignore the full story told by the data. They ignore the relationships between data measures that further inform the optimal staffing for a medical practice.

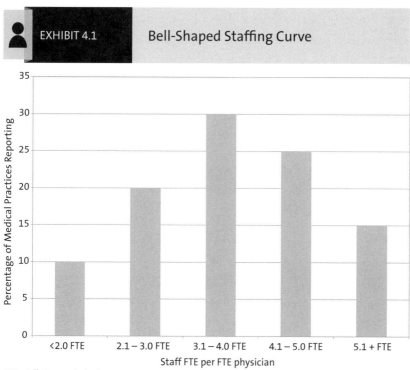

EXHIBIT 4.1   Bell-Shaped Staffing Curve

FTE = Full-time equivalent

Lesson 4: Relationship Between Data Measures

When we combine different measures in a graph, we are able to see
relationships between each measure. In the case of staffing a medical
practice, what we really want to learn is the level of staffing needed
to optimize quality, profitability, practice efficiency, and patient
satisfaction. It is through the impact of one data element on another
that we can begin to learn about optimal staffing levels in a medical
practice. Let's examine the relationship between staffing and productivity and staffing and profitability.

Staffing to Optimize Productivity

The data demonstrate that there is a relationship between staffing and productivity. Exhibit 4.2 is a scatter plot that helps us learn the relationship between these two data elements. The number of staff FTE per FTE physician is reported on the x, or horizontal, axis and the number of procedures per FTE physician is reported on the y, or vertical, axis. A regression line is also demonstrated in this exhibit. A regression line allows us to look at the path of the center of the data so that conclusions may be drawn from the relationship between FTE support staff per FTE physician and productivity. In this case the regression line increases from left to right in the exhibit, suggesting

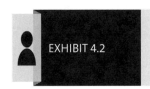

| EXHIBIT 4.2 | Impact of Total FTE Support Staff per FTE Physician on Total Procedures per FTE Physician in All Multispecialty Groups |

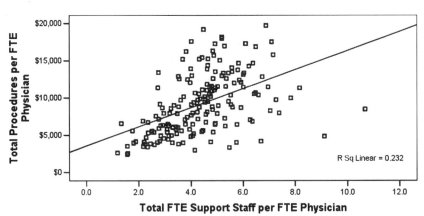

MGMA Cost Survey: 2010 Report Based on 2009 Data

Data reprinted with permission from: Medical Group Management Association. *Cost Survey for Multispecialty Practices: 2010 Report Based on 2009 Data*. Englewood, Colo.: Medical Group Management Association.

that there is a positive relationship between the increase in staff and the increase in productivity for a medical practice.[1]

In fact, not only does productivity increase with the number of FTE staff per FTE physician as demonstrated in Exhibit 4.2, but also when we examine the relationship between FTE staff per FTE physician and revenue and the relationship between FTE staff per FTE physician and operating expenditures, revenue and expenditures tend to increase with the number of FTE staff per FTE physician. This suggests that there are significant benefits, as well as costs, to higher staff FTE levels.

Staffing to Optimize Profitability

In Exhibit 4.3 we use this same approach to identify the number of staff that the most profitable practices have and the number of staff reported for those medical practices that are the least profitable. The x-axis reflects total FTE support staff per FTE physician. The y-axis reflects total medical revenue after operating cost per FTE physician — a measure of practice profitability. The regression line also increases from left to right in this exhibit.

The data suggest that there is a relationship between staffing levels and profitability. This finding is important. Staff costs typically represent more than 30 percent of the total medical revenue that is earned in a medical practice. This is surpassed only by another human resource cost, that of providers (both physicians and non-physician providers). Consequently, the number, skill mix, and assignment of the staff are critical in terms of the overall profitability of a medical practice.

---

[1] The author acknowledges the work of David N. Gans, MHSA, FACMPE, of MGMA who has worked tirelessly to analyze data in MGMA's various datasets and translate the data into information that can be used by a medical practice to improve business and operating performance.

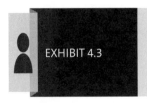

EXHIBIT 4.3

Impact of Total FTE Support Staff per FTE Physician on Total Medical Revenue After Operating Cost per FTE Physician in All Multispecialty Groups

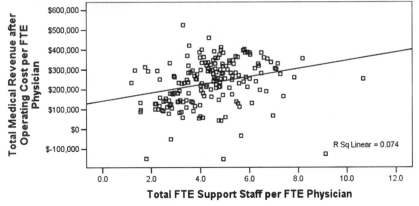

MGMA Cost Survey: 2010 Report Based on 2009 Data

Data reprinted with permission from: Medical Group Management Association. *Cost Survey for Multispecialty Practices: 2010 Report Based on 2009 Data*. Englewood, Colo.: Medical Group Management Association.

By analyzing staffing levels and medical practice profitability together, we learn that:

> ➤ Typically, the more staff in a medical practice, the greater the level of profitability in the practice (the increase in revenue associated with the increased productivity exceeds the higher staff cost), but

> ➤ Overall, there is a weak relationship between the number of staff and practice profitability.

This suggests that the impact on profitability is not necessarily the result of having more staff but rather of having the right staff doing the right things that are contributing to practice profitability.

> The impact on profitability is not necessarily the result of having more staff but rather of having the right staff doing the right things that are contributing to practice profitability.

Lesson 5: Staffing in Better-Performing Medical Practices

We have conducted extensive studies of the data and the relationships between data elements in "better-performing" medical practices. For this discussion, the criteria for the selection of better-performing medical practices are financially based, as opposed to those that may have better quality or better patient care outcomes. Financial performance has been selected because it is more objective than other measures when differentiating performance among medical practices. For purposes of staffing, the financial measures also get to the heart of the business-of-medicine concerns related to staffing strategies in a medical practice.

We have learned three key staffing insights from the experiences of better-performing medical practices:[2]

➤ *Insight 1:* Better-performing medical practices tend to have a higher quantity of staff. They have more staff on a per-FTE-physician basis than their practice counterparts.

➤ *Insight 2:* The cost of staff on a per-FTE-physician basis is also higher. This could be due to a number of factors: (1) they have more staff, (2) the staff are paid higher wage rates, and/or (3) they have a different skill mix of staff.

---

[2] Better-performing medical practices have been isolated from the MGMA datasets due to their higher performance in the areas of (1) profitability and cost management; (2) productivity, capacity, and staffing; or (3) accounts receivable and collections.

In short, we know that staffing costs are higher for better-performing medical practices.

➤ *Insight 3:* The real insight we gleaned from better-performing practice data is that although these groups have more staff and a higher cost of staff on a per-FTE-physician basis, many of these medical practices actually have lower staff costs on a percentage of total medical revenue basis. This is an exciting finding! It means that better-performing practices are reaping the benefits of their higher staffing levels and higher cost on a per-FTE-physician basis by having the staff devoted to the right things that increase profitability in the medical practice. Even though the cost of staff on a per-FTE-physician basis is higher in our better-performing practices, the cost of staff as a percentage of total medical revenue is lower. Better-performing medical practices ensure that staff are performing at optimal levels, making a positive contribution to practice profitability.

These insights are summarized in Exhibit 4.4.

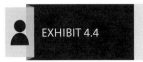

EXHIBIT 4.4	Insights from Better-Performing Practices

Better-performing practices:

Insight 1   Have more staff

Insight 2   Have a higher cost of staff on a per-FTE-physician basis

Insight 3   Tend to have lower staff cost as a percentage of total medical revenue

Translating the Data to Usable Information

What do these lessons mean for a typical medical practice? First, a medical practice that simply cuts staff is not going to achieve long-term, sustainable financial performance. Why? When staff are cut below the level necessary to run an effective and efficient practice, there is waste. One key category of that waste is physicians being asked to perform nonclinical tasks. In fact, some estimate that up to 60 percent of the activities conducted by physicians can be delegated to another qualified person in the medical practice. You need the right number of staff and the right skill mix of staff devoted to the right activities in a medical practice to provide the infrastructure and support to the billable provider to achieve high levels of profitability and performance.

Second, it is important that we correctly staff our medical practices. The data suggest that staffing is linked to both productivity and practice profitability, so we have to get it right.

STAFF BENCHMARK DATA

With this discussion as background, let's look at the staff benchmark data that are available for us as we determine whether a medical practice has the "right staff."

Exhibit 4.5 outlines the staffing data that are included in MGMA's annual survey instruments. The benchmark data available on staffing are reported in three main survey instruments published by MGMA:

➤ *Cost Survey for Single-Specialty Practices*

➤ *Cost Survey for Multispecialty Practices*

➤ *Performance and Practices of Successful Medical Groups*

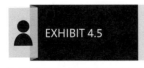

| EXHIBIT 4.5 | Staff Benchmark Data |

Staff Category	Staff Function
Business operations staff	General administrative Patient accounting General accounting Managed care administrative Information technology Housekeeping, maintenance, security
Front office support staff	Medical receptionists Medical secretaries, transcribers Medical records Other administrative support
Clinical support staff	Registered nurses Licensed practical nurses Medical assistants, nurse aides
Ancillary support staff	Clinical laboratory Radiology and imaging Other medical support services

Source: Medical Group Management Association. *Cost Survey for Single-Specialty Medical Practices* and *Cost Survey for Multispecialty Practices.* Note: These are standard definitions used each year. Reprinted with permission.

In the left column of the exhibit are four main categories of staff that are reported in the benchmark dataset. The four categories are:

Business operations: Business and administrative staff

Front office: Staff involved in pre- and postvisit activities

Clinical support: Staff involved in the clinical services provided by the medical practice

Ancillary: Staff involved in clinical laboratory, imaging, and other similar services

The right column of the exhibit expands each staff category into specific job functions. The benchmark data are provided at both levels in the survey instruments: job category and job function. For example, in the category of clinical support staff, the data are reported separately for each function: registered nurses (RNs), licensed practical nurses (LPNs), and medical assistants (MAs), and also summarized in one category as total clinical support staff.

The following sections outline the four key staffing benchmarks that are used by medical practices to evaluate their staffing levels.[3]

Benchmark 1: Staff FTE per FTE Physician

This benchmark reflects the number of full-time equivalent (FTE) staff in comparison with the number of FTE physicians in the medical practice. By full-time equivalent, we mean the number of staff and physicians that you consider in your medical practice to be full-time. Note that this definition varies among medical practices. For example, some medical practices consider a 35-hour workweek to be full-time, while others consider full-time as a 40-hour workweek. This definition is left up to each medical practice.

Calculation: The benchmark of staff FTE per FTE physician is reported as a ratio. For example, if the data report 5.00 FTE support staff and 25.00 FTE physicians, the ratio is calculated as 5 divided by 25, or .20 FTE. If your staff consistently incur overtime, be sure to include this in the benchmarking analysis. For example, if Nurse Betty reports 10 hours of overtime each week, that is an FTE equivalency of .25 FTE. Isolated overtime does not need to be incorporated into the benchmarks; however, routine overtime should be included to recognize the true staffing volume in a medical practice.

The benchmark staff FTE per FTE physician essentially represents a macrolevel comparison between medical practices of the same

---

[3] The benchmark data from MGMA are cited in this book. Please see the Additional Resources section for these and other benchmark sources.

specialty to provide early identification of potential opportunity to alter the staffing levels or staffing deployment model in a medical practice. Note that we are saying "potential opportunity," because we need to "peel back the onion" and move to a more detailed analysis to determine whether there is true opportunity to change staffing patterns in a medical practice.

The data for staff FTE per FTE physician are reported at the specialty level. In some specialties, the data are also reported separately depending on whether the medical practice is considered a physician-owned practice or whether it is owned by a hospital or integrated delivery system.

In Exhibit 4.6 we provide an example of the data available by specialty for the staff FTE per FTE physician benchmark. Please note that this is an example only. The actual benchmark data that should be used are the most current benchmark survey instrument and the dataset that most closely resembles your medical practice (for example, peer medical practices of the same specialty or peer medical practices of the same specialty and the same ownership type).

Benchmark 2: Staff FTE per FTE Provider

A variation of the staff FTE per FTE physician benchmark is to compare the ratio of staff FTE to the FTE of all providers, to include not only physicians, but also nonphysician providers. A medical practice that employs nurse practitioners or physician assistants should analyze staff FTE on a per FTE provider basis in addition to staff FTE per FTE physician.

This benchmark is also available in the dataset and is defined as staff FTE per FTE provider. By evaluating staff FTE per FTE provider, we recognize the staffing needs that are required to support all providers (physicians and nonphysicians) in a medical practice.

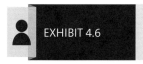

EXHIBIT 4.6	**Staff FTE per FTE Physician**

Staff Category	Staff FTE per FTE Physician
General administrative	.25
Patient accounting	.65
General accounting	.05
Managed care administrative	.05
Information technology	.10
Housekeeping/maintenance/security	.10
Total Business Operations Staff	**1.10**
Medical receptionists	1.00
Medical secretaries/transcribers	.15
Medical records	.30
Other administrative support	.15
Total Front Office Support Staff	**1.65**
Registered nurses	.35
Licensed practical nurses	.40
Medical assistants, nurse aides	.95
Total Clinical Support Staff	**1.60**
Clinical laboratory	.35
Radiology and imaging	.25
Other medical support services	.20
Total Ancillary Support Staff	**.65**
Total Employed Support Staff	**4.55**

Note: Totals will not sum; example of median data is reported.

Calculation: The benchmark of staff FTE per FTE provider is reported as a ratio. For example, if the data report 5.00 FTE support staff and 30.00 FTE providers (including physicians and nonphysician providers), the ratio is calculated as 5 divided by 30, or .17 FTE.

In addition to benchmarking the quantity of staff, the skill mix of staff in a medical practice can be benchmarked. This is done by viewing the benchmark at the functional level, which helps a medical practice determine whether it has the right type of staff devoted to key functions. For example, in the area of clinical support staff, we compare a medical practice's clinical support staff at the categorical level, which is the total clinical support, and at the functional level, which involves peeling back the onion and comparing the mix of registered nurses, licensed practical nurses, and medical assistants in the practice. In each of these instances, we use the benchmark that is published for staff FTE per FTE physician (or per FTE provider). The difference only relates to the level by which we evaluate staffing, that is, whether it is by staff category (the total of all staff in the category, such as total clinical support staff) or staff function (the specific work functions or skill mix of the staff, such as RN, LPN, and MA).

Benchmark 3: Staff Cost per FTE Physician

Benchmark data are also available for analyzing staffing costs in a medical practice. One key benchmark is staff cost per FTE physician. This helps you determine whether the cost of your staff is in line with peer practices.

Calculation: This benchmark is reported at a dollar level and is calculated as staff cost divided by FTE physicians in the practice. For example, if the cost of staff is $100,000 in a medical practice and there are 5.00 FTE physicians, the calculation would be $100,000 divided by 5, or $20,000 per FTE physician.

To determine whether your clinical support staff cost is in line with comparable medical practices, first calculate your cost on a per-FTE-physician basis and then compare it using the benchmarking survey data. Data are also available for each staff category and staff function. An example of this type of benchmarking data is provided in Exhibit 4.7.

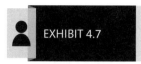

EXHIBIT 4.7   Staff Cost per FTE Physician

Staff Category	Staff Cost per FTE Physician
General administrative	$18,920
Patient accounting	$20,155
General accounting	$3,400
Managed care administrative	$3,000
Information technology	$5,600
Housekeeping/maintenance/security	$2,900
Total Business Operations Staff	**$45,300**
Medical receptionists	$25,500
Medical secretaries/transcribers	$4,950
Medical records	$7,125
Other administrative support	$4,500
Total Front Office Support Staff	**$42,450**
Registered nurses	$15,750
Licensed practical nurses	$13,000
Medical assistants, nurse aides	$26,700
Total Clinical Support Staff	**$57,800**
Clinical laboratory	$11,600
Radiology and imaging	$11,500
Other medical support services	$10,000
Total Ancillary Support Staff	**$26,400**
Total Employed Support Staff	**$154,500**

Note: Totals will not sum; example of median data is reported.

Benchmark 4: Staff Cost as a Percentage of Total Medical Revenue

In our earlier discussion regarding better-performing practices, we learned that staff cost as a percentage of total medical revenue is actually lower for many better-performing medical practices. To determine if the cost of your staff — the overhead that is attributed to staff in your medical practice — is consistent with benchmark data, first calculate your staff cost. Then compare this cost to the total medical revenue generated in your medical practice.

This, too, can be carried out at the level of staff category and staff function. In this way, you can determine whether the overhead costs associated with staff in your medical practice are higher or lower than in other medical practices and identify areas where you might have cost-saving opportunity related to staff.

Calculation: The benchmark is reported as a percentage. As an example, if your staff cost is $100,000 and total medical revenue for the practice is $300,000, the ratio is calculated at .33. In this example, 33 percent of total medical revenue is devoted to staffing cost. Exhibit 4.8 presents an example of the benchmarking data that are available for staff cost as a percentage of total medical revenue.

Additional Staff Benchmarks

In addition to these four benchmarks, which are commonly used to identify opportunity to improve your staffing model, there are a number of others that also can be used.

These include staff FTE per output of work:

> ⇒ Staff FTE per total relative value unit (TRVU)
> ⇒ Staff FTE per work relative value unit (WRVU)
> ⇒ Staff FTE per patient

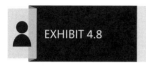

EXHIBIT 4.8 Staff Cost as a Percentage of Total Medical Revenue

Staff Category	Staff Cost as a Percentage of Total Medical Revenue
General administrative	2.55%
Patient accounting	2.60%
General accounting	.40%
Managed care administrative	.40%
Information technology	.70%
Housekeeping/maintenance/security	.35%
Total Business Operations Staff	**6.40%**
Medical receptionists	3.60%
Medical secretaries/transcribers	.60%
Medical records	.90%
Other administrative support	.75%
Total Front Office Support Staff	**6.50%**
Registered nurses	2.20%
Licensed practical nurses	1.85%
Medical assistants, nurse aides	3.55%
Total Clinical Support Staff	**8.00%**
Clinical laboratory	1.25%
Radiology and imaging	1.50%
Other medical support services	1.20%
Total Ancillary Support Staff	**3.50%**
Total Employed Support Staff	**23.75%**

Note: Totals will not sum; example of median data is reported.

There are also staff benchmarks based on staff FTE per input of work: specifically, staff FTE per square feet of the medical practice.

Definitions for each measure are provided in the following sections.

Staff FTE per Total RVU or per WRVU

The staffing needs in a medical practice vary based on the actual work that is performed in the practice. Staff benchmark data are reported for both total relative value unit (RVU) and work RVU, which are medical practice production "outputs." The WRVU has been determined to be the closest unit of measure of physician work. It reflects both work quantity and type of service provided to the patient. Some medical practices have developed their own internal targets for staffing, utilizing the practice expense RVU; however, benchmark data are not yet available for this measure.

Calculation: This benchmark is expressed as a ratio and is calculated as follows: staff FTE divided by total RVU or work RVU.

Staff FTE per Patient

Another benchmark based on production output is staff FTE per patient. Staff are a step-fixed cost to a medical practice. That is, at some point an increase in patient volume signals the need for additional staff to be hired over current levels for certain work functions.

Calculation: The benchmark is expressed as a ratio and is calculated as follows: staff FTE divided by the number of patients.

Staff FTE per Square Feet

The larger the medical practice, the more staff that are needed. This benchmark recognizes an input to the practice — the square footage of the practice's facility. Simply walking around the medical practice consumes valuable staffing resources and time. In addition, a medical practice with multiple practice sites will have more staff than a medical practice with a single site, with a full complement of staff required to support the internal patient flow process at each practice location.

Calculation: The benchmark is expressed as a ratio and is calculated as follows: staff FTE divided by square feet of the medical practice's facility.

More sophisticated medical practices often use these additional benchmarks to refine their analysis and often develop staffing targets based on these measures. For example, a medical practice site may be able to increase staffing levels only when a targeted staff FTE per WRVU is achieved.

Benchmarking Comparison of Multiple Practice Sites

The benchmarks can also be used to analyze the differences in staffing strategies for multiple practice sites within an organization. An example of this benchmarking is reported in Exhibit 4.9. The fundamental question that needs to be asked is, why? Why are the practice sites different? It may be that there are legitimate reasons for the differences in staffing related to the specialty, the type of work performed, and the work quantity. However, it also may be that the staffing deployment models have migrated over time and it is now time to realign staffing with the work throughout the organization.

In this figure, practice site A has a one-to-one assignment of a registered nurse to each 1.00 FTE physician. At site B, there is a combination of each type of clinical support staff; however, this site has more licensed clinical staff than the benchmark. The last site (site C) has an overall greater number of clinical staff per FTE physician compared with the other two practice sites, and it is higher than the benchmark. This is an excellent starting point for the analysis of clinical support staff for each care site. The next step is to evaluate physician productivity and the type of work delegated to the staff at each site.

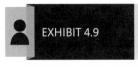

	Multisite Comparison of Staffing Levels: Staff FTE per FTE Physician
EXHIBIT 4.9	

Job Function	Site A	Site B	Site C	Benchmark
Registered nurse	1.00	.50	.50	.35
Licensed practical nurse	0.00	.50	.50	.40
Medical assistant	0.30	.50	1.00	.95
Total clinical support staff	**1.30**	**1.50**	**2.00**	**1.60**

Note: Benchmark column will not total; sample median data is reported.

BENCHMARK LIMITATIONS

Staff benchmarking data help you determine where your medical practice may have staffing opportunity. However, these data should not be used as absolute targets or goals absent an understanding of the benchmark limitations.

Four examples are provided here that showcase the limitations to the benchmarks that need to be taken into account when interpreting the data. The purpose of drawing your attention to the benchmark limitations is to ensure that once you have benchmarked the staffing levels in your medical practice, you can translate the data to usable information in order to take action and improve your staffing model.

> ➤ *Work tasks.* Though the benchmark data are reported at the level of the job function, such as receptionist or registered nurse, it is not possible from these data to identify the specific work tasks that have been delegated to the staff. For example, a medical practice with a streamlined patient scheduling system will have fewer staff than a medical practice with a

cumbersome scheduling process. So, a medical practice that offers advanced access where patients simply phone in and are slotted for a same-day appointment will typically have fewer staff than a medical practice that requires the schedulers to take messages or obtain nurse approval for the same-day appointment. The work is less streamlined and less efficient in this latter practice.

As another example, the front office staff of two medical practices may perform very different work. In one medical practice, the staff may be required to manage inbound telephone calls, conduct insurance verification and benefits eligibility, collect time-of-service payments, print orders, and prepare medical records and forms. In another medical practice, the work of the check-in staff may be limited to verifying demographic and insurance information and collecting time-of-service payment. These two medical practices will have very different staffing levels, with the former likely having more front office staff due to the additional work tasks. If these two practices have the same staffing complement, the second medical practice will likely have staff with significant capacity.

➢ *Technology.* The benchmark data have not been segmented relative to the level of technology used in a medical practice. For example, if a medical practice has a Web portal through which patients request appointments, request prescription renewals, obtain test results, and pay their bills, typically, fewer staff are required to manage the inbound telephone calls when compared with a medical practice that does not offer patients electronic access. As this example illustrates, the use and leverage of technology dramatically affects staffing levels.

➢ *Productivity.* Staff levels in a medical practice represent a step-fixed cost, that is, as the practice becomes more productive, at some point more staff are needed to manage the work volume. The issue of productivity is only indirectly addressed by the benchmark data (for example, by analyzing staff costs as a percentage of total medical revenue). Staff volumes vary depending on the workload of the medical practice. The definition of this workload varies based on the type of work being performed. For example, a determination of the appropriate number of staff to manage the telephones is dependent on the volume of inbound telephone calls. Similarly, a determination of the appropriate number of staff to assist the physician during the clinical visit is dependent on the number of patient visits and the actual work that is delegated to the nurse or medical assistant to perform. Thus, a medical practice with high productivity will typically have more, not fewer, staff to assist with its work, and it is difficult to discern the variability in work productivity inherent in the staff benchmark data.

➤ *Number of practice sites.* As medical practices set up satellite sites throughout a community, they typically must hire additional staff to work at the sites (unless the staff travel from site to site). Thus, a medical practice that has developed a geographic distribution strategy throughout its community will likely have more staff than a practice that is based at only one site. Although the benchmark survey instruments report the number of practice sites in the entire dataset for the specialty (data are reported by quartile, including 25th percentile, median, 75th percentile, and 90th percentile), the direct contribution of these additional sites to the benchmark data is not evident. We typically observe that medical practices with a number of satellite sites have more staff than their peers and, in some cases, less productive staff. This is due to the fact that a core cadre of staff is needed to staff the satellite site regardless of patient volume levels, thereby negatively impacting the ability of the medical practice to take advantage of economies of scale.

Thus, there are significant limitations to the staff benchmark data. The staff benchmarks that were discussed earlier in this chapter do not permit the level of distinction related to work tasks delegated to staff, the use and leverage of technology, practice productivity, and number of practice sites, in particular. However, the staff benchmarks are effective in identifying areas of opportunity in staffing that require further analysis.

> There are limitations to the benchmark data. Despite these limitations, benchmarking staff levels and costs to peer practices helps to identify opportunities for improvement.

BASIC APPROACH TO STAFF BENCHMARKING

The benchmarking process is simple and straightforward. First, identify the key work functions that you have asked your staff to perform. Then identify the hours typically needed by the staff to perform these functions each week to derive an FTE level that is devoted to each function. This information is the baseline from which you are able to then benchmark a host of indices related to the quantity, skill mix, and cost of your staff.

For example, let's say you have Bob working the check-in desk and medical assistant Sally retrieving and rooming patients, and they both work full-time (in this example, a 40-hour workweek) in the medical practice. Exhibit 4.10 reflects the hours per week and the FTE devoted to each of these work functions.

 EXHIBIT 4.10 Basic Benchmarking Example

Name	Work Function	Hours per Week	FTE
Bob	Medical reception	40	1.00
Sally	Medical assistant	40	1.00
Total		80	2.00

Of course, the staffing patterns in many medical practices tend to be a bit more complicated than this example. At times, Bob may also perform medical records functions and, at times, Sally may be assigned to manage scheduling. If this is the case, simply approximate the hours per week that each staff member devotes to specific work functions in the practice. As demonstrated in Exhibit 4.11, Bob and Sally now have new work functions and FTE designations, given their multitasking assignments, though their total FTE will remain the same at 1.00 FTE each and the total staff FTE for the practice (in this case, 2.00 FTE) remains unchanged.

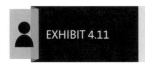

| EXHIBIT 4.11 | Basic Multitasking Benchmarking Example |

Name	Work Function	Hours Per Week	FTE
Bob	Medical reception	30	.75
	Medical records	10	.25
Subtotal		**40**	**1.00**
Sally	Medical assistant	20	.50
	Medical reception	20	.50
Subtotal		**40**	**1.00**
Total		**80**	**2.00**

Note: By mapping the work functions to the survey instrument, Bob is reported as .75 FTE medical reception and .25 FTE medical records. Sally is now reported as .50 FTE medical reception and .50 FTE medical assistant.

In the example in Exhibit 4.11, Bob typically devotes 30 hours per week to medical reception functions involved in the patient check-in process and 10 hours per week to medical records functions. He is now categorized as .75 FTE medical reception (calculated as 30 hours divided by a 40-hour workweek) and .25 FTE medical records (calculated as 10 hours divided by a 40-hour workweek). On the other hand, Sally typically divides her time between medical assisting activities and scheduling, devoting about 20 hours each week to each of these functions. In her case, she is now reclassified as .50 FTE medical assistant and .50 FTE medical reception, as scheduling is one of the tasks included in the survey operational definition for medical receptionists (calculated as 20 hours divided by a 40-hour workweek for each of her primary job functions).

We apply this process to each staff member in the medical practice. The work function listed for each staff is the one that most closely matches the operational definitions provided in the benchmark survey instrument. In our benchmarking example, Sally's role as a scheduler is mapped to the benchmarking survey for the work function of medical reception. The result is the baseline data that are needed to compare staffing levels in a medical practice to available benchmarks.

Continuing with our benchmark example, let's assume there are three physicians who work full-time in the medical practice in which Bob and Sally work. The staff FTE per FTE physician is calculated in Exhibit 4.12 and is reported as a ratio.

EXHIBIT 4.12	Calculating Staff FTE per Physician FTE		
Key Work Functions	**Staff FTE**	**Physician FTE**	**Staff FTE per FTE Physician**
Medical reception	1.25	3.00	.42
Medical records	.25	3.00	.08
Medical assistant	.50	3.00	.17
Total	**2.00**	**3.00**	**.67**

This ratio, staff FTE per FTE physician, is typically the first benchmarking analysis that is conducted to determine if there is staffing opportunity in a medical practice. Using the example in Exhibit 4.12, we compare the total staff level of .67 FTE per FTE physician with the benchmarks for total staff FTE per FTE physician for similar medical practices. We then look at the specific categories of the staff and compare the subtotals at the categorical level with the benchmarks (for example, the category of total clinical support staff). Finally, we expand the categorical level to the work function level and use this to also compare staff levels (for example, registered nurses, licensed practical nurses, and medical assistants — the work functions that are added together to create the categorical level of total clinical support staff).

By benchmarking staff to both the categorical and functional staffing levels, we move beyond the overall number of staff FTE per FTE physician or per FTE provider to recognize the roles and skill mix of the staff. At each level we take a "deeper dive" into identifying potential staffing opportunity in comparison to peer medical practices.

BENCHMARKS AND STAFF COSTS

Now that we have benchmarked the quantity of staff and the skill mix of staff in the medical practice, we turn to the cost of staff and the benchmarks that are available for this analysis. There are two key benchmarks available for staffing cost analysis: (1) staff cost per FTE physician, and (2) staff cost as a percentage of total medical revenue.

By benchmarking staff costs in a medical practice, you are able to determine if you are paying more or less for staff in comparison to the benchmarks (defined as staff cost per FTE physician). More importantly, you can determine if your medical practice overhead that is devoted to staffing costs is in line with other medical practices (defined as staff cost as a percentage of total medical revenue).

Continuing with our basic benchmarking example, to benchmark staff cost per FTE physician, first identify the salary for each staff member and then assign that salary based on FTE to each of the staff member's work functions. This is reported in Exhibit 4.13.

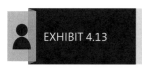

EXHIBIT 4.13 — Staff Cost per Work Function

Name	Total Salary	FTE per Work Function	Salary per Work Function
Bob	$28,000	.75 medical reception .25 medical records	$21,000 $ 7,000
Sally	$32,000	.50 medical assistant .50 medical reception	$16,000 $16,000
Total	**$60,000**	**2.00 FTE**	**$60,000**

Then assign the cost on a per-FTE-physician basis. Assuming that three physicians work in this medical practice, divide the salary per work function by 3.00 FTE physicians. This is reported in Exhibit 4.14. As demonstrated by the data, overall staff cost per FTE physician is $20,000, with $12,333 assigned to medical reception, $2,333 assigned to medical records, and $5,333 assigned to medical assistant functions. Once these data are computed for the medical practice, compare the data to available benchmarks to measure the cost per work function per FTE physician against peer practices.

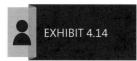

EXHIBIT 4.14 — Staff Cost by Work Function per FTE Physician

Work Function	Staff Cost	Staff Cost per FTE Physician
Medical reception	$37,000	$12,333
Medical records	$ 7,000	$ 2,333
Medical assistant	$16,000	$ 5,333
Total	**$60,000**	**$20,000**

Finally, compare the cost of staff as a percentage of total medical revenue to peer practices. Continuing with our example, let's suppose that the three physicians generate $500,000 in medical revenue. In this basic example, total staff cost as a percentage of total medical revenue is calculated as 12 percent ($60,000 divided by $500,000). Once this is calculated, take a deeper dive into the data and compare staff cost as a percentage of total medical revenue at the staff category and work function levels to the benchmarks. This tells you whether the amount of overhead attributed to staff based on staff category and work function is more or less than similar medical practices.

SUMMARY

In this chapter, we discussed the important relationships among different measures. In particular, there appears to be a relationship between profitability and staffing levels in a medical practice. Better-performing medical practices tend to have more staff and they have higher staffing costs, yet staff cost as a percentage of total medical revenue is lower than their counterparts. This suggests that to appropriately staff a medical practice, you need the right staff doing the right things — no more, no less.

We also shared the basic steps in benchmarking staff in a medical practice. These include benchmarking the quantity of staff, the skill mix of staff, and the cost of staff. By benchmarking the staff in your medical practice to peer practices, you learn areas of potential opportunity to improve your staffing levels and staff models. It is important to identify the skill needs of staff involved in medical practice work functions with the goals of matching staff to the required work function and ensuring expected levels of productivity and performance.

Because there are limitations to the staff benchmark data, we continue our quest to learn where we may have opportunity to improve the staffing strategy in the medical practice. In the next chapter we evaluate the current workload of the staff and compare this to expected staff workload ranges. By utilizing both staff benchmarks and expected workload ranges, you have the data needed to answer the question, "Do I have the right staff in my medical practice?"

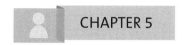

CHAPTER 5

The Staff Workload Evaluation Process

The use of expected staff workload ranges is a more precise measure of staffing opportunity. They take into account the actual work and work volume that is performed by the staff.

—Deborah Walker Keegan, PhD, FACMPE

We have now benchmarked the staffing levels and costs in the medical practice. Through the benchmarking process we have identified potential areas of opportunity to improve the staffing model. We recommend that these areas of opportunity receive the initial focus as we now work to refine our staffing analysis by comparing the staff's work quantity with expected workload ranges.

In this chapter, we describe:

- ➤ The importance of staffing for the work
- ➤ Expected staff workload ranges for key work functions
- ➤ Limitations to expected staff workload range data
- ➤ The basic process to evaluate staff workload and tasks
- ➤ How to interpret staff workload range data
- ➤ How to use expected staff workload ranges to identify required staff resources

IMPORTANCE OF STAFFING FOR THE WORK

Although benchmarks are important and are used as one method for determining whether a medical practice is staffed correctly, as we discussed in Chapter 4, there are very real limitations to the benchmarks. The actual workload and tasks that have been delegated to staff in a medical practice are not recognized in the benchmarking process. Similarly, if two medical practices have the same number of staff, yet the patient visit volume is dramatically different, there may also be staffing opportunity, as one of the practices may have more (or fewer) staff than needed to manage this patient visit volume. Ideally, we want to staff for the actual work that is performed in a medical practice. The use of expected staff workload ranges helps us analyze staffing levels by taking into account the type of work and quantity of work performed by the staff.

EXPECTED STAFF WORKLOAD RANGES FOR KEY WORK FUNCTIONS

Expected staff workload ranges are available for each key step in the patient flow and business processes of a medical practice.[1] The expected staff workload ranges were derived by sitting with staff at their desks and observing the approximate time staff take to perform each of their key work functions. The workload ranges are based on a seven-hour productive day in the medical practice.

> There are different staff workload ranges depending on the type of work that has been delegated to the staff to perform.

---

[1] For more information on staff workload ranges, see Woodcock, Elizabeth W. 2009. *Mastering Patient Flow: Using Lean Thinking to Improve Your Practice Operations, 3rd Edition,* Englewood, Colo., Medical Group Management Association, and Walker Keegan, Deborah; Elizabeth W. Woodcock; and Sara M. Larch. 2009. *The Physician Billing Process: 12 Potholes to Avoid in the Road to Getting Paid* Englewood, Colo.: Medical Group Management Association.

It is important to recognize that each medical practice uses different work processes. For example, the steps needed to check in a patient at one medical practice will differ (often greatly) when compared with another medical practice. As another example, a medical practice that has been able to leverage technology at high levels will be more efficient than one that is still working with manual or paper systems. Thus, expected staff workload ranges are rather broad, and each medical practice needs to validate whether the range is appropriate and consistent for its specific situation. By comparing the current workload of the staff to expected workload levels, we begin to understand the variation in staffing that may have been created in a medical practice due to the work processes that have been delegated to the staff to perform.

There are different staff workload ranges depending on the type of work that has been delegated to the staff to perform. For example, if a staff member assigned to work patient check-in is responsible for validating information, conducting insurance verification, and obtaining time-of-service payments, the expected workload range for this staff member (the total amount of patients the staff member is able to check in) is lower when compared with a staff member who is only tasked with verifying information at the time a patient presents to the office.

As another example, the type of inbound telephone call determines the time needed to respond to the caller and the skill mix needed for the staff to manage the call. A scheduling call, for example, typically takes longer than a call that involves simply transferring the caller to the appropriate party. Similarly, a nurse triage call typically involves more time than either scheduling or call transfer and it also involves a different skill set (in this case, a nurse instead of a telephone operator or scheduler). Exhibits 5.1 through 5.4 report the expected staff workload ranges for each key step in the patient flow process:

➤ Telephone management and scheduling (see Exhibit 5.1)

➤ Front office, including registration, check-in, check-out, referral management (see Exhibit 5.2)

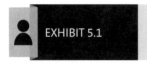

| EXHIBIT 5.1 | Expected Staff Workload Ranges for Telephone Management and Scheduling |

Work Function	Per Day	Per Hour	Per Transaction
Telephones with messaging*	300–500	42–71	N/A
Telephones with routing (electronic system) only*	1,000–1,200	142–171	N/A
Appointment scheduling with no registration*	75–125	11–18	N/A
Appointment scheduling with full registration†	50–75	7–11	N/A
Insurance verification via Website†	N/A	N/A	1–3 minutes
Insurance verification via telephone call†	N/A	N/A	2–10 minutes
Benefits eligibility via Website†	N/A	N/A	3–10 minutes
Benefits eligibility via telephone call†	N/A	N/A	5–20 minutes

N/A = not applicable

*Source: Woodcock, Elizabeth W. 2009. *Mastering Patient Flow: Using Lean Thinking to Improve Your Practice Operations*. Englewood, Colo.: Medical Group Management Association. Reprinted with permission.

†Source: Walker Keegan, Deborah; Elizabeth W. Woodcock; and Sara M. Larch. 2009. *The Physician Billing Process: 12 Potholes to Avoid in the Road to Getting Paid*. Englewood, Colo.: Medical Group Management Association. Reprinted with permission.

➤ Visit and clinical support, including telephone nurse triage and patient flow (see Exhibit 5.3)

➤ Billing and collections, including charge entry, payment posting, insurance account follow-up, and patient account follow-up (see Exhibit 5.4)

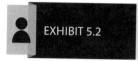

EXHIBIT 5.2 **Expected Staff Workload Ranges for Front Office**

Work Function	Per Day	Per Hour
Registration with insurance verification (on-site or previsit)	60–80	9–11
Patient check-in with registration verification only	100–130	14–19
Patient check-in with registration verification and cashiering only	75–100	11–14
Check-out with scheduling and cashiering	70–90	10–13
Check-out with scheduling, cashiering, and charge entry	60–80	9–11
Referrals (inbound or outbound)	70–90	10–13

Source: Walker Keegan, Deborah; Elizabeth W. Woodcock; and Sara M. Larch. 2009. *The Physician Billing Process: 12 Potholes to Avoid in the Road to Getting Paid.* Englewood, Colo.: Medical Group Management Association. Reprinted with permission.

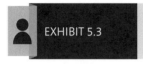

| EXHIBIT 5.3 | Expected Staff Workload Ranges for Visit and Clinical Support | |

Work Function	Per Day	Per Hour
Telephone nurse triage*	65–85	8–12
Patient intake: patient rooming, vital signs	Variable based on specific work that can be delegated; typically, 25 to 40 patients per day	N/A
Visit support: Nurse visit support, procedures, education	Variable based on specific work that can be delegated; typically, 25 to 40 patients per day	N/A
Health and wellness coaching	Variable, based on type of coaching provided; see Chapter 12: Staffing the Medical Home Model for a detailed discussion	N/A

N/A = not applicable

Note: The expected staff workload range assumes full nurse triage and advice, not simply prescription renewals or responding to inquiries of a nonclinical nature, such as scheduling or information requests.

*Source: Woodcock, Elizabeth W. 2009. *Mastering Patient Flow: Using Lean Thinking to Improve Your Practice Operations.* Englewood, Colo.: Medical Group Management Association. Reprinted with permission.

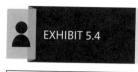

Work Function	Per Day	Per Hour
Charge entry line items without registration	375–525	55–75
Charge entry line items with registration	280–395	40–55
Payment and adjustment transactions posted manually	525–875	75–125
Insurance account follow-up, research and resolve by phone	N/A	6–12
Insurance account follow-up, research and resolve by appeal	N/A	3–4
Insurance account follow-up, check status of claim and rebill	N/A	12–60
Patient account follow-up	70–90	10–13

N/A = not applicable

Source: Walker Keegan, Deborah; Elizabeth W. Woodcock; and Sara M. Larch. 2009. *The Physician Billing Process: 12 Potholes to Avoid in the Road to Getting Paid*. Englewood, Colo.: Medical Group Management Association. Reprinted with permission.

The "Potholes" book contains additional expected staff workload ranges related to billing; the above exhibit reports a subset of this data.

We will use these data in the exhibits in the following chapters as we discuss innovative staffing strategies for each of these work functions in the medical practice.

LIMITATIONS TO EXPECTED STAFF WORKLOAD RANGE DATA

There are two important limitations to using expected staff workload range data in determining a staffing strategy for a medical practice. First, the workload ranges only relate to the *quantity* of work, not the *quality* of work that is performed. Staff are not robots, and day-to-day practice operations are not always routine; that is one reason why we have assumed only a seven-hour productive day. When validating or determining an expected workload range, however, it is important to recognize that when there are questions regarding quantity versus quality, quality needs to trump quantity each and every time. That is, you may need to relax the expected workload ranges for your particular staff if quality is not at the expected level.

> Staff are not robots, and day-to-day practice operations are not always routine. Quality needs to trump quantity each and every time.

Second, the ability to perform within these workload ranges may vary due to internal practice-specific factors such as your facility, technology, and the specific processes that the staff have been tasked to perform. Some medical practices have adopted streamlined processes, while others are more encumbered with more process steps, process hand-offs, and other similar complexities. Hence, it is important to verify that the expected staff workload range is consistent with your specific medical practice.

If your staff are performing at lower workload ranges than expected levels, you may have an opportunity to learn from others and import the best practices of other medical groups, or you may have an opportunity to innovate your work processes via technology. In contrast, if your staff are performing at higher workload ranges than expected levels, yours could be a "best" practice or it could suggest the need to evaluate work quality to ensure it is at its level best.

BASIC PROCESS TO EVALUATE STAFF WORKLOAD AND TASKS

The process of comparing current staff workload levels with those of the expected workload ranges is relatively straightforward.

1. *Determine the unit of work.* First, determine the unit of work for a particular job function. For example, in the case of a staff member assigned to telephone management, the unit of work is the inbound telephone call volume. In contrast, in the case of a staff member assigned to support the patient flow process, the unit of work is patient visit volume.

2. *Evaluate the expected staff workload range and modify it for your medical practice.* Review the staff workload range for each work function and ensure that the expected range is generally consistent with your medical practice's experience. If not, modify the expected staff workload range for your medical practice.

3. *Measure the current work volume of staff.* Measure the current work volume of the staff in the medical practice using a representative week. You do not want to measure the workload at extreme highs and lows. Other staffing strategies can be used to manage high and low peak work periods.

4. *Analyze performance gaps.* Finally, compare this work volume with the expected workload range to identify staffing opportunity related to work levels.

Case Study

Let's proceed through these steps to evaluate staff workload by using an example related to patient check-in.

1. *Determine the unit of work.* The unit of work for patient check-in is the number of patients who are checked in each day. In most medical practices, one staff member devoted to this function can check in 100 to 130 patients per day

if the work involves simply verifying information with
the patient (as outlined in Exhibit 5.2). The staff workload
ranges are based on a seven-hour productive day. This
means that, on average, patient check-in takes 3.2 to
4.2 minutes per patient.

2. *Evaluate the expected staff workload range and modify it for your
medical practice.* To effectively use the expected workload
range in your medical practice, first determine if the time to
perform that work function is consistent with your medical practice's experience. Do this by evaluating the average
time it takes for a staff member to conduct this work in your
medical practice. Ask the staff to record the times for patient
check-in by patient for a one-week period or sit with the
staff and observe the average time it takes them to complete
check-in processes. For this example, let's assume that the
expected workload range of 100 to 130 patients per day is
consistent with that observed at the medical practice. Let's
further agree that we want to take a conservative approach
and use 100 patients per day to analyze the quantity of
work conducted by the current staff.

3. *Measure the current work volume of staff.* In step three, determine the patient check-in volume at your medical practice.
The unit of work is the patient visit volume presenting for
appointments. Exhibit 5.5 reflects the patient visit volume
by day of the week for our sample medical practice.

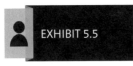

| EXHIBIT 5.5 | Patient Visit Volume by Day of the Week |

Day of Week	Mon	Tue	Wed	Thu	Fri
Visit Volume	200	150	100	75	35

4. *Analyze performance gaps.* Analyze the performance gaps in step 4 by calculating the staff full-time equivalent (FTE) levels required for the current work volume. Do this by dividing the visit volume by the expected workload level — in this example, 100. For example, on Monday, the visit volume is 200 patients. Divide that by 100 to learn that 2.00 FTE are required to manage this work volume. Proceed in a similar fashion for each day of the week.

After calculating the required FTE for the work volume, report the current FTE assigned to the work. In our sample medical practice, let's assume there are 2.00 FTE assigned to patient check-in. The final step is to calculate the gap, which is defined as required FTE less current FTE.

Exhibit 5.6 reflects these calculations. As demonstrated by the exhibit, on Monday our sample medical practice has an appropriate number of staff assigned to the work. Throughout the rest of the week, however, there is increasing capacity for the staff assigned to this work function, given the decline in patient visit volume each day of the week.

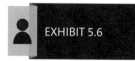

| EXHIBIT 5.6 | Required FTE for Patient Visit Volume and Performance Gap | | | | |

Day of Week	Mon	Tue	Wed	Thu	Fri
Visit volume	200	150	100	75	35
Required FTE	2.00	1.50	1.00	.75	.35
Current FTE	2.00	2.00	2.00	2.00	2.00
Gap	0.00	.50	1.00	1.25	1.65

HOW TO INTERPRET STAFF WORKLOAD RANGE DATA

If you learn that the quantity of work that is performed by your staff is significantly different from the expected range (as we did in the previous example), ask and address the question, why?

> By comparing actual work levels, you are in a better position to determine whether you have the right number of staff devoted to a particular work function and task.

If staff are performing at lower productivity levels than expected, potential reasons could include:

> ➤ The staff are highly multitasked and not able to perform this and their other responsibilities, and/or

> ➤ Work processes are highly encumbered, thereby creating inefficiencies

If staff are performing at higher productivity levels than expected, potential reasons could include:

> ➤ Operational innovations may have permitted the staff to outperform other practices, and/or

> ➤ The work quality may not be at the expected level

By comparing actual work levels, you are in a better position to determine whether you have the right number of staff devoted to a particular work function and task. By comparing the workload levels currently handled by your staff to the expected staff workload ranges, important questions are raised that should be considered when evaluating your staffing levels. For example:

> ➤ Why are staff performing at levels that vary from the expected range?

> ➤ Is our work process streamlined or encumbered?

➤ Is there a better way to carry out this process?

➤ Is there opportunity to improve performance and outcomes?

HOW TO USE EXPECTED WORKLOAD RANGES TO IDENTIFY REQUIRED STAFF RESOURCES

Another way to use expected staff workload ranges is to identify the number of staff required to perform a certain project, function, or task. For example, a medical practice may decide to focus the telephones in a central call center. By utilizing the expected staff workload ranges, we can begin to identify the number of staff required to meet patient telephone demand.

As an example, let's assume that the medical practice receives 1,500 telephone calls per day, with one third of the calls involving patient scheduling, one third requiring messages to be taken, and one third relating to clinical issues. Let's also assume that the medical practice wants to include nurse triage staff on the telephones to manage the clinical calls. In this scenario, we analyze the data and employ the expected staff workload ranges, as demonstrated in Exhibit 5.7.

This example shows that this sample medical practice will generally need to staff its new patient access center with 7.00 FTE telephone schedulers/message staff and 7.50 FTE nurse triage staff (assuming the midpoint of the calculated ranges). As described in Chapter 7, Staffing the Telephones, we recommend a further refinement of the data to identify the actual staff needed by day of week, session per day, and time of day, as well as to take action to reduce inbound telephone demand. However, this example demonstrates the valuable use of expected staff workload ranges to identify staffing levels required to carry out specific work functions.

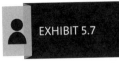

EXHIBIT 5.7	Using Expected Staff Workload Data to Identify Staff Volume		

Call Volume, 1,500 inbound calls	Call Type	Expected Workload Range, Calls per Day	Number of Staff FTE Required
500 calls	Appointment scheduling with no registration	75–125	4.00–6.67
500 calls	Message-taking	300–500	1.00–1.67
Total Scheduling/ Message Staff			**5.00–8.34**
500 calls	Nurse triage	65–85	6.67–8.33
Total Nurse Triage Staff			**6.67–8.33**

Source: Expected workload range data are derived from Exhibit 5.1, Expected Staff Workload Ranges for Telephone Management and Scheduling and Exhibit 5.3, Expected Staff Workload Ranges for Visit and Clinical Support. Reprinted with permission.

The use of expected staff workload levels also helps you diagnose staffing challenges in your medical practice. Let's say, for example, that a staff member devoted full-time to patient check-in can be expected to check in 100 patients per day. Based on a seven-hour productive day, this means 14 patients per hour, or 4 minutes and 20 seconds for each patient. It is Monday morning in the medical practice, and at 8:30 a.m. 20 patients present at the same time to be checked in by this one staff member. What do we already know about the staffing strategy of this medical practice? Not only will patients be queued up for long periods of time, but there will also be a significant delay in getting the patients roomed and ready for the physician. A static staffing model — staffing at the same level throughout the day regardless of patient visit volume — fails to take into account the actual work that physically can be done by a single staff member within a specific time period. (This concept of creating variable staffing deployment consistent with the work is one of the themes of this book — staff for the work — and is further discussed in Chapter 13, Staffing Models for Fluctuating Work Levels and Other Realities.)

SUMMARY

As we discussed in this chapter, it is important to not only benchmark staffing levels to survey instruments, but also to evaluate the current workload of the staff and compare it with expected workload ranges. Through these two approaches — staff benchmarking and staff workload comparison — you are able to identify opportunity related to staffing volumes and skill mix of staff. Armed with these data, you can then answer the question, "Do I have the right staff?," and identify whether there is staffing opportunity in your medical practice.

We now turn to the second key question: "Are the staff doing the right things?" The chapters that follow describe innovative staffing strategies for each key function inherent in the patient flow process, including staffing for telephones, front office, the visit, medical records, and billing. In addition, we present staffing strategies for the day-to-day realities of a medical practice — the fluctuating work volume that occurs on particular days or sessions per day. We also present innovative staffing strategies to meet the changing healthcare and reimbursement environments, to include staffing for electronic health records, consumer-directed health plans, and medical home models of care. Making sure that the staff are doing the right things is critical if we seek to optimize our care team.

PART 3

Are the Staff Doing the Right Things?

Innovative Strategies for Key Work Functions

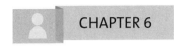

CHAPTER 6

Creating a Care Team

Effective teams have a culture that fosters openness, collaboration, teamwork, and learning from mistakes.

—Crossing the Quality Chasm:
A New Health System for the 21st Century

Today the typical worker is doing knowledge and service work in a highly competitive environment that requires innovation and relies on collective achievement of work results.

—Leveraging the New Human Capital: Adaptive Strategies,
Results Achieved, and Stories of Transformation

In healthcare, a patient-centered care team is a prerequisite for success. In medical practices, we grapple not only with the complex human biological form, but also with the emotional elements associated with health and healing. This requires a well-orchestrated approach to each facet of the patient flow process. It also requires compassion and empathy. It is no longer good enough that the patient is treated as if he or she is just a diagnosis or patient number 152 of the day. As you design your care team, you need to ensure that the patient is at the center of your care processes.

In addition, we are piling more and more work on the physicians. Asking them to work harder and faster is not the answer. You need a fully engaged care team to meet the healthcare needs of your patient population.

In this chapter, we:

➤ Define a high-performing care team

➤ Review action to create a high-performing care team

➤ Discuss the special needs of small, large, and academic medical practices

WHAT IS A HIGH-PERFORMING CARE TEAM?

The traditional staffing model in a medical practice has placed the physician at the center of all the activity, with each staff member revolving around this center, preferably in a well-coordinated fashion. However, this is not the reality for most medical practices. Instead of a well-coordinated team, we often witness turf battles between the front and back offices, misunderstandings regarding roles and responsibilities, some staff who work hard while others shirk their responsibilities, and other similar acts, reminiscent of dysfunctional families. The telephones are ringing off the hook; there is paper, paper, and more paper everywhere (even though we are supposedly paperless or paper sparse); communication channels and avenues are simultaneous and often loud; the pace is hectic, and everyone is stressed to the max — only to go home and wake up the next day and do it all over again.

Many medical practices have become complacent. There is nothing new going on. Each and every day staff come into work and attempt to work the same old processes and the same old systems that have been in place, often for decades.

> Imagine a new staffing strategy with the patient at the center of the care team.

The traditional staffing model in a medical practice with the physician at its center is depicted in Exhibit 6.1.

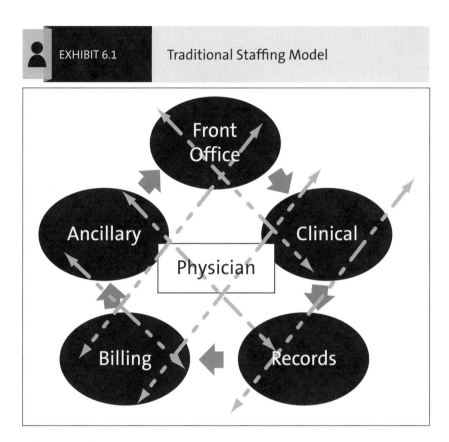

EXHIBIT 6.1 Traditional Staffing Model

Front Office

Ancillary

Clinical

Physician

Billing

Records

High-Performing Care Teams

Imagine a new staffing strategy with the patient at the center of the care team. Work processes are designed to meet the patient's needs and there is systematic workflow around the patient. This does not mean that there are no idiosyncratic events that occur in a medical practice. Every day we are faced with new situations and challenges regarding patients and their care. But it does mean that staff are connected to their roles and provide exceptional service and clinical delivery in a well-coordinated fashion. There are no surprises for the patients and patients don't have to learn how to maneuver convoluted work processes. They don't have to "go fish" for information. The care team anticipates what the patient needs and takes the care and service to the patient.

A high-performing team in a medical practice places the patient at the center of the team (Exhibit 6.2). By placing the patient at the center of the team, you can then design work processes from a patient perspective. Once the processes are patient-centric, a physician-led, well-coordinated care team can do the rest. In a high-performing care team, the support staff have a common, overarching focus to meet the health and care needs of the patient.

Leading this central patient focus are physicians. Support staff are highly functional and integrated, with well-rehearsed and orchestrated roles and assignments. Process and patient handoffs, from one task to the next, are minimized. Patient wait time is minimized. In short, the physician leads a highly functional and well-coordinated care team that is whole-heartedly focused on patient care and support. Importantly, in today's medical practices, the care team is often asked to extend across the continuum of care. For example, a care manager may work with a patient to facilitate transitions of care from primary care to specialty care to hospital care to home care. Thus, members of the care team need to not only be internally focused on patients, colleagues, and co-workers, but also need to be externally focused on the delivery system itself.

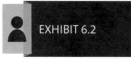

EXHIBIT 6.2   Patient-Focused High-Performing Team

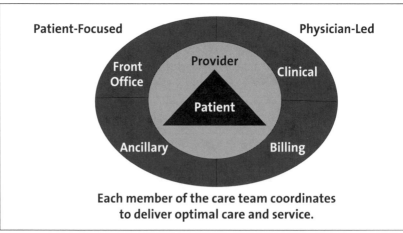

Patient-Focused   **Physician-Led**

Front Office   Provider   Clinical

Patient

Ancillary   Billing

**Each member of the care team coordinates
to deliver optimal care and service.**

With physicians and staff working together to focus on the patient, evaluate work processes to determine whether the process has been designed for the patient. In many cases, you may discover that the work process is in reality designed for a specific physician or a specific staff member or group of staff rather than the patient. Examples include:

> Patients must wait two weeks to obtain a referral

> Patients must wait seven days for a test result that is ready in two days

> Patients are required to contact the office 48 hours in advance of prescription renewal

> Scheduling calls go to voice mail

> Telephone calls are transferred to the answering service at lunch

> There are specific times to call the medical practice to schedule an appointment

> An automated attendant system is "out of numerical order"; for example, press 5 for this and 1 for that

> The office is closed on Wednesday afternoons (with no instruction to patients as to what to do if they happen to be ill on a Wednesday afternoon)

> Few providers are in the practice on Friday afternoons, limiting same-day access opportunity

By placing the patient at the center of the care team, you can begin to analyze current work processes and redesign them to streamline the work and better meet patient needs and wants. (See Chapter 16, Work Process Redesign, for a stepwise approach to redesigning work processes.) A difficult task to be sure, but those medical practices that recognize that the patient is truly the leading customer are able to break down the silos and hierarchies, dismantle old systems and processes, and redesign the delivery system to improve value to patients and their families.

CREATING A HIGH-PERFORMING CARE TEAM

Teamwork results from institutionalizing the values of the medical practice, developing clear performance expectations, providing training and development opportunities, and providing ongoing assessment of behavior in the context of the medical practice's expectations. In essence, you want your team to "become who we are" not "what we want to be." The work of teamness should be inherent in what the staff do, not be set aside as a special project.

It is important to avoid the "five dysfunctions of a team."[1] They include absence of trust, fear of conflict, lack of commitment, avoidance of accountability, and inattention to results. The following actions help avoid these dysfunctions and create a high-performing care team for your medical practice:

- Design patient flow processes through a patient lens
- Articulate teamwork expectations
- Evaluate staff on teamwork
- Involve staff in information and decisions and create a sense of ownership
- Immediately address "killer phrases" that deflate the team
- Emphasize "us" versus "me"
- Provide support to the team so that members can do their very best work
- Be a relentless example of teamwork

Each of these actions is now described.

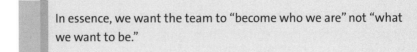

In essence, we want the team to "become who we are" not "what we want to be."

---

[1] Lencioni, Patrick. 2002. *The Five Dysfunctions of a Team: A Leadership Fable*. San Francisco: Jossey-Bass; p. 188.

Design Patient Flow Processes Through a Patient Lens

Evaluate each of your patient flow processes through a patient lens. This can be done by asking patients to participate in focus groups or meetings to review the process from their perspective. It can also be done by asking staff to evaluate a particular process using a patient lens and then report what works and what improvements they recommend and why (with these recommendations shared with patients for their feedback). In this way, the staff are actively engaged in analyzing processes and making recommendations as part of the team to improve process performance.

Articulate Teamwork Expectations

Define the type of team you want for your medical practice, then employ a self-assessment instrument for staff to evaluate their level of teamwork. For example, team behaviors that are often articulated in a medical practice include:[2]

- Meets and exceeds patient expectations for care and service
- Exercises good judgment and initiative
- Actively participates on the team
- Works with others to achieve consensus
- Contributes knowledge to the team
- Conducts objective problem-solving
- Demonstrates interpersonal effectiveness
- Supports other team members
- Fosters trust and respect
- Develops mutual accountability for the work
- Is creative and innovative
- Is positive, with high energy and engagement

---

[2] Walker, Deborah. 1999. "Laying the Foundation for Continual Change: Teaming for Innovation," pp. 19-30. In Key, M.K.: *Managing Change in Healthcare: Innovative Solutions for People-Based Organizations*. New York: Healthcare Financial Management Association, McGraw-Hill. Adapted from Team Self-Assessment Instrument, p. 29.

Once you have developed teamwork expectations, ask the staff to evaluate themselves regarding each of these attributes as part of a self-assessment. The supervisor or manager should then provide perspective regarding the staff member's strengths and areas of opportunity to improve team-oriented behaviors.

Evaluate Staff on Teamwork

One expectation for a care team is to actually have staff who care. Patients expect to be treated with compassion and empathy. Yet, we have often run into staff who are not at all compassionate and not at all empathetic. Instead, these staff are "me"-oriented and appear unable to extend warmth and caring. You have probably met one or more of these staffers at some point in your career. There are many examples of problematic behavioral styles; here are just a few:

- The work revolves around them; "it's all about me"
- Patients are not welcomed to the practice; the staff act as though the patients are an interruption
- The patient is treated as if he or she is a number or a disease, not a person
- The staff tell patients what they can't do and do not try to identify what can be done
- The staff gripe most of the time about the work they have to do
- The staff always have an excuse when patients complain about their service
- The staff member is not a "morning person"
- The staff are not customer-friendly, in fact, some are not even people-friendly

Staff who are not able to demonstrate this most basic of human emotions — empathy — for patients have no place in a medical practice. Compassion and empathy are very difficult to teach. Faced with two job applicants, neither of whom possess the requisite knowledge and teamwork skills, it may be necessary to recruit based on culture and behavior and train for the work or task, rather than the other way around.

To ensure that staff are focused on teamwork and to reinforce that you truly expect team-oriented performance, the talent management process and any incentive or bonus plans that are developed for your medical practice should also focus on teamwork. We discuss both of these areas further in Chapter 19, Talent Management: Nurse Betty Behaving Badly, and Chapter 20, Staff Compensation and Incentive Plans.

> Share as much financial and operational information as possible with your team.

Involve Staff in Information and Decisions and Create a Sense of Ownership

A mistake that is frequently made in a medical practice is to withhold information from the staff (or not actively share information). This is a mistake, because through data and information we can expand the breadth and scope of knowledge of the staff, which will permit them to assist in self-management and identify new work processes. After all, the best person to recommend a change to the work functions and tasks is the person who has been working those functions and tasks, often for many years, and is closest to and owns the process.

Share as much financial and operational information as possible with your team. This includes bringing staff up to date on the changing healthcare environment and asking for their assistance in continually scanning the environment, both the external environment (to learn about changes in the community, for example), and the internal environment (for example, their own workload and work processes). In this fashion, they become active contributors to the medical practice. Through these actions, you begin to transition staff from employee to partner, one who has a sense of ownership and pride in the work and work product and makes a true contribution to the team.

Staff should also regularly be shown the results of their work. For example, a staff member who is assigned to conduct insurance account follow-up should know their days' revenue outstanding, their accounts receivable greater than 90 days, and their net collection rate, as well as the targets and goals that are expected of their performance. In this fashion, the team member can self-manage and initiate course corrections, if appropriate.

> Through these actions, you begin to transition staff from employee to partner, one who has a sense of ownership and pride in the work and work product and makes a true contribution to the team.

Immediately Address Team "Killer Phrases"

Killer phrases are those silver-tongued bullets that some staff offer up on a regular basis. These phrases zap the energy of other staff in the medical practice and create obstacles to moving the organization forward. Examples of killer phrases include:

- It won't work
- We've tried that before
- It will mean more staff
- There's not enough time to do that, too
- Who thought that one up?
- Don't go there…
- It's not in the budget
- It's not in my job description
- They won't let us
- Yes, but…

Let staff know that you do expect them to raise issues and concerns, but at the same time, you expect recommended solutions to the problems. And don't let the killer phrases stand; instead, push back. For example, if a staff member says "we tried that before," ask when was it tried, what were the assumptions, what resources were applied, what was the outcome, and what lessons were learned? As another example, if the staff say "it is not in the budget," ask the staff to identify what resources are needed, what savings in other areas could be considered, and how could it be performed without incurring high expenditures? In this way, staff are not able to simply criticize or voice (often loudly) their lack of support. Instead, their job is to share their talent and actively contribute to the team.

Emphasize Us Versus Me

Ask staff to put on a team hat when they provide input and advice. They then transition from a focus on "me" to a focus on "us." Help staff maintain this focus. Whenever staff talk about what they want, ask them to put it into terms that relate to the patient and to the team. In this way, your medical practice can begin to move from an individual focus ("it's all about me!") to a team focus.

Provide Support to the Team so that Members Can Do Their Very Best Work

The role of the leader is to keep each individual focused on his or her strengths and help each team member perform at his or her best. Everyone has weaknesses. If we focus only on the weakness, we fail to capitalize on staff members' strengths.[3] Develop work functions, tasks, and tools that are specific to team members and aligned with their capabilities.

---

[3] Peter Drucker stressed the importance of focusing on employee strengths, rather than their weaknesses, and the importance of aligning work consistent with employee strengths. (Per classroom discussion.)

Be a Relentless Example of Teamwork

The physician and practice executive should epitomize the teamwork that is expected of the staff. This can be done in the following ways:

- Hold same-day huddles with the staff to review the day and discuss what worked and what did not work from the day (or morning) before

- Share practice data and information and ask staff for input to improve

- Stay calm and exercise a focused determination on improving patient health and wellness

- Treat every person on the care team as an equal; no one person or one type of staff should be viewed as more important than the other

- Expect more from staff; challenge staff to think critically and assign work to staff that stretches their comfort zones

- Say "please" and "thank you"[4]

SPECIAL NEEDS OF SMALL MEDICAL PRACTICES

In small medical practices, the team may consist of two or three staff who are often multitasked to do many jobs in the practice. The medical assistant may also manage patient check-in or the patient check-in staff may also be the person who performs patient check-out and manages the telephones. It is important in a small medical practice to recognize this expanded work scope by helping the staff understand day-to-day priorities and exercise flow in the work they perform.

For example, if a staff member is seated at the front desk and is on the telephone with a patient, and a patient enters to check in for his or her visit, the staff member needs to learn how to manage the

---

[4] Peter Drucker identified the lack of common courtesy in today's corporations and advocated simple courtesies to improve the work environment. (Per classroom discussion.)

face-to-face visit with the patient. Institute role playing to help the staff learn how to remain calm while at the same time providing nonverbal cues to the patient who enters the suite, thereby acknowledging the patient's presence and importance. Juggling the two priorities is difficult, and it should not be assumed that a staff member understands how to perform this dual role.

SPECIAL NEEDS OF LARGE MEDICAL PRACTICES

In large medical practices, managers and supervisors have a particular challenge in directing and overseeing the work of the care team. With large staff units, we often witness a "moral hazard." It is easy for a staff member to shirk responsibilities and not pull his or her weight on the team. It is also easy for a staff member's strengths to be overlooked and his or her needs not to be met. In these instances, consider dividing up the staff into smaller units, with a lead, supervisor, or manager working with a smaller number of staff so that they can provide the support and tools needed for the staff to succeed and can also identify areas of opportunity to educate and counsel staff as appropriate.

SPECIAL NEEDS OF ACADEMIC PRACTICES

Academic practices, with their expanded role in research and education, can be particularly challenging when it comes to solidifying a care team. Residents in training typically are required to hold a continuity-of-care clinic, which means that residents in each of their years of training have their own patients assigned to them. Each year, however, there is a migration of residents when the senior residents graduate and the first-year residents join the team. The patient who is followed by a resident should have a seamless experience during the resident's annual migration.

To solve this problem, many academic practices establish a team approach to care. For example, in a resident continuity-of-care clinic, there might be three teams: A, B, and C (or a team color or name). Each team has an attending physician, two to four residents, a licensed nurse, two medical assistants, and a scheduler. When a patient calls the medical practice, he or she selects the team from the list of automated attendant options and the call is directed to the appropriate team. When residents graduate, the patient stays within the same team and continuity of care continues, with each resident advancing one year in his or her training but staying active in the patient's care. Such a strategy also works with nonacademic medical practices that have a plethora of part-time physicians. Continuity of care should be seamless for the patient, with a care team designated to meet patient needs.

SUMMARY

In this chapter, we shared the definition of a patient-centered, physician-led team. We also reviewed actions that can be taken to create and strengthen your care team. A care team that is truly caring should be a core competency of all medical practices. By adopting specific actions and tools, a medical practice is able to transition staff from being simply employees to being active, contributing members of the care team. This is an important distinction and one that high-performing medical practices have been able to achieve. This is not a panacea. That is, you will still have days when things don't go as expected and you will still have staff who at times exhibit outlier behavior. However, you can begin the difficult process of transforming the culture of your medical practice to a physician-led, high-performing care team. "The dual focus employee, whose knowledge or service work requires mind and heart as well as hands, is the new human capital."[5]

---

[5] Burud, Sandra, and Marie Tumolo. 2004. *Leveraging the New Human Capital: Adaptive Strategies, Results Achieved, and Stories of Transformation*. Palo Alto, Calif.: Davies-Black Publishing.

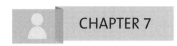

CHAPTER 7

Staffing the Telephones

I can't believe the scheduling calls go to voice mail! Do they even want me as a patient?

—Anonymous Patient

Patients report general dissatisfaction with their ability to reach their physician via the telephone. In some medical practices, the telephone management process is indeed broken; the telephone rings off the hook or worse, goes to voice mail, and the calls are a constant interruption to the day-to-day operations of the practice. Many medical practices have solved their telephone dilemma by recognizing the importance of telephones as a patient access channel and staffing the telephones with the same careful attention that they pay to staffing for the visit.

In this chapter, we:

- ⇒ Discuss the importance of telephone management
- ⇒ Measure and analyze inbound telephone demand
- ⇒ Provide performance expectations for telephone management
- ⇒ Build a successful staffing model to manage telephone demand
- ⇒ Share innovative staffing strategies for telephone management
- ⇒ Provide key questions to address as you staff the telephones

IMPORTANCE OF TELEPHONE MANAGEMENT

Although many medical practices are expanding their use of Web portals, secure message threads, and other electronic access methods, the telephone is still the technology typically used by patients, referring physicians, hospitals, nursing homes, pharmacies, and other stakeholders to contact the medical practice. Accessing the medical practice by telephone is considered the external patient flow process. Correct staffing of the telephones is critical for the financial viability of a medical practice; over the telephone, we typically learn the patient's demographic and insurance information to permit us to bill for rendered services, obtain required referrals, and know what payment to collect from the patient at the point of care. The telephones are a pathway through which patients access needed care services and medical advice.

TRADITIONAL TELEPHONE MANAGEMENT PROCESS

The traditional process for call management is depicted in Exhibit 7.1. In the traditional telephone management process, a medical practice uses an automated attendant for inbound calls, with the caller selecting from a menu of options. For example, patients select 1 to schedule an appointment, 2 to talk to a nurse, and so forth. Telephone calls are managed by telephone operators/schedulers who schedule the patient for a visit, transfer the call to an appropriate party, or take a message (either manually or electronically). The majority of messages relate to clinical issues, and the messages are typically transmitted to the nurse in the back office area for resolution.

This traditional call management process is costly and encumbered. We often hear complaints by patients, physicians, and staff. Some of the common complaints are listed in Exhibit 7.2.

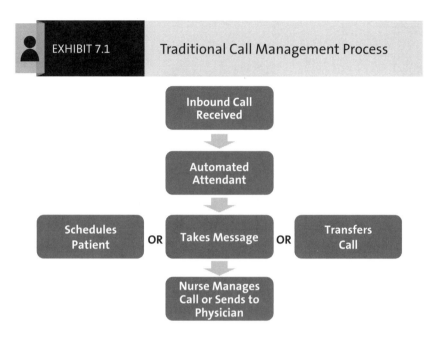

EXHIBIT 7.1 Traditional Call Management Process

Inbound Call Received

Automated Attendant

Schedules Patient OR Takes Message OR Transfers Call

Nurse Manages Call or Sends to Physician

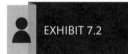

EXHIBIT 7.2 Common Complaints Regarding Telephone Management

Area	Performance Problem
People	Inconsistent skill set Poor customer service Inconsistent information provided to patient Inaccurate scheduling
Messages	Insufficient message detail Inconsistent scripting with patient Incomplete reason for visit Unrealistic turnaround times provided to patients
Work processes	Long wait time on-hold Delays in returning calls to patients Telephone tag with patient for call-back Each call touched more than once

> The traditional call management process for a medical practice is costly and encumbered.

These complaints can be resolved with appropriate staffing strategies, which include:

- ➤ The correct number of staff assigned to manage telephones
- ➤ The correct skill mix of staff assigned to the phones
- ➤ Performance expectations regarding service and care
- ➤ Performance expectations regarding call turnaround time
- ➤ Consistent, standard work processes
- ➤ Education and scripting

PERFORMANCE EXPECTATIONS FOR TELEPHONE MANAGEMENT

It is important to institute performance expectations for telephone management and to measure your staff's ability to achieve these standards. Exhibit 7.3 outlines some common expectations regarding telephone management to help you get started.

Metrics to Measure Telephone Management

There are a number of metrics that can be tracked related to inbound telephone calls and telephone management of those calls. Exhibit 7.4 lists the type of data that are routinely available to assess appropriateness of a medical practice's staffing model devoted to the volume of calls and performance of telephone management.

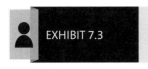

EXHIBIT 7.3 Performance Expectations for Telephone Management

Measurement	Standard
Abandonment rate	Less than 5 percent for each day and period
Average time to answer	Within three rings
Maximum time on hold	Two minutes
Compliance with scripts	100 percent
Turnaround time for calls	Urgent and same-day appointment requests: 30 minutes
	Clinical questions, nonurgent: Same day for calls received before 4:00 p.m.; next business day for calls received after 4:00 p.m.
	R_x renewals: Direct patients to pharmacy; one business day
	Test results: Provide patients with expectation during visit or at check-out; one business day after test result/ interpretation received
	Referrals: one business day
	All calls acknowledged within two hours of receipt regardless of ability to fully answer the request
Message accuracy	98 percent accuracy for spelling, grammar, completeness
Reason for visit	98 percent accuracy for completeness; ability to use reason to prepare for visit

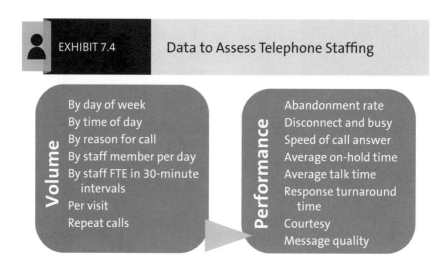

EXHIBIT 7.4   Data to Assess Telephone Staffing

Volume
- By day of week
- By time of day
- By reason for call
- By staff member per day
- By staff FTE in 30-minute intervals
- Per visit
- Repeat calls

Performance
- Abandonment rate
- Disconnect and busy
- Speed of call answer
- Average on-hold time
- Average talk time
- Response turnaround time
- Courtesy
- Message quality

To build the staffing model for telephones (see the following section), use the first three volume measures: inbound calls by day of week, inbound calls by time of day, and inbound calls by reason for call. The selection of these measures is not to suggest that the other measures are not useful. Indeed, these and other measures help to determine the magnitude of opportunity available to improve telephone management in a medical practice. In fact, many of the measures serve as early warning signals that the process is broken.

Some of the measures help refine the staffing strategy for telephone management once it is adopted. For example, the volume of calls managed within 30 minutes by each staff member helps identify potential performance gaps among staff. Staff may be spending too long on the telephone attempting to manage the patient's inquiry and perhaps need further education and training. Alternatively, some staff may be cutting the call short and are not able to gauge the patient's full needs to take a complete and accurate message.

BUILDING THE STAFFING MODEL FOR TELEPHONE MANAGEMENT

Follow the four steps first presented in Chapter 3 to optimize the staffing deployment model for telephone management.

1. *Benchmark staff full-time equivalents (FTEs) and costs.* Operational definitions in the survey instruments describe the type of staff included in each of the job categories and job functions for which benchmark data are reported. In the case of telephone staff, these map to medical receptionists in the survey instrument for those staff who are involved in scheduling and telephone messaging. For calls taken by clinical support staff, use the RN, LPN, or MA work functions, depending on the licensure of staff involved in telephone management. Follow the steps outlined in Chapter 4, The Staff Benchmarking Process, to benchmark staff FTEs and costs.

2. *Evaluate staff workload.* Follow the steps in Chapter 5 to analyze staff workload and compare it to expected workload ranges. The unit of work is the inbound telephone volume managed by the staff. Identify the appropriate staffing levels required to manage the volume and type of call. Recognize variation in inbound telephone demand by day of week and time of day and perform a gap analysis, comparing current staffing levels with those suggested by the workload evaluation analysis.

3. *Redesign work processes.* Determine the preferred work process to manage inbound telephone calls for your practice. This may include a redesign of the work process, a co-location of staff in the medical practice, and/or a change to staff roles and responsibilities.

4. *Innovate your model.* Create a flexible staffing model rather than a static model of staffing in order to staff for the work consistent with the variability in inbound telephone demand.

We now demonstrate each of these steps using data from our sample medical practice.

Step 1: Benchmark Staff FTEs and Costs

Follow the steps outlined in Chapter 4 to benchmark your staff FTEs and staff costs for telephone management to the benchmark. Telephone staff who conduct scheduling and message-taking are reported under the MGMA Cost Survey category of "total front office staff" and under the job function of "medical receptionists." Per the MGMA survey definitions, the job function category of medical receptionists includes switchboard operators, schedulers, and appointment staff.[1]

Nurses who manage telephone triage and advice are reported under the MGMA Cost Survey category of "total clinical support staff" and under the job function consistent with their licensure — RN, LPN, or MA.

Step 2: Evaluate Staff Workload

The unit of work for telephone staff is the volume of inbound telephone calls and the type of inbound calls that are managed by the staff.

In step 2, first evaluate the volume of inbound calls by day of week and time of day. To obtain inbound telephone call volume, determine whether your telephone system or vendor is able to provide this information. If not, simply ask the staff to collect these data for a one-week period. The goal is to obtain a representative sample of data. The staffing model can be adjusted over time based on feedback from other performance measures. For example, if call abandonment

---

[1] Operational definitions are reported in each of the MGMA survey instruments. This operational definition is consistent across all of MGMA's survey instruments. Copyright MGMA. Reprinted with permission.

rates are higher than baseline, then the staffing model may need adjustment. Similarly, if a new physician is hired who generates a significant increase in inbound telephone demand, an adjustment to the staffing model may be needed. A staffing model is not static; it is regularly evaluated and updated consistent with the changing needs of a medical practice.

Once you have obtained the inbound telephone call volume by day of week and time of day, graph this information to learn more about the data. Exhibit 7.5 reflects a sample of the telephone volume by day of week for our sample medical practice. From these data we learn that more staff are needed to work the telephones on Monday, tapering off throughout the week. This is not at all surprising for most medical practices; inbound telephone demand is often highest on Mondays. The key to staffing the telephones is to staff for this work variability in call demand by day, not simply create a static staffing model that is the same throughout the entire week, regardless of inbound telephone call volume.

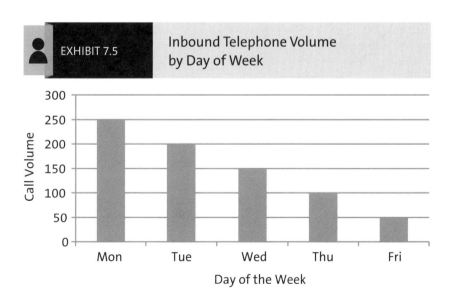

EXHIBIT 7.5   Inbound Telephone Volume by Day of Week

Also graph the inbound telephone calls by time of day. In Exhibit 7.6, we can see that the inbound telephone call volume also varies by time of day. Calls at our sample medical practice are at their highest volume from 8:00 a.m. to 12:00 p.m. each day. In fact, approximately 70 percent of the calls are received in the morning between these hours. Thus, we learn from these data that more staffing resources need to be deployed in the morning than in the afternoon, again suggesting the use of a flexible rather than static staffing model to manage the inbound telephone demand.

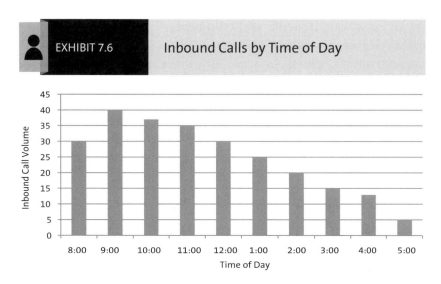

EXHIBIT 7.6   Inbound Calls by Time of Day

A further refinement to the staffing model can be made by linking both measures we have examined thus far: inbound telephone calls by day of week and time of day. For example, you may find that your call volume is highest on Monday mornings between 8:00 a.m. and 10:00 a.m. Additional refinements can be made for seasonality (for example, flu season) and other variations, such as open enrollment for health insurance or the call volume two days after patient statements are mailed. In this fashion, you are staffing for the work.

Beyond the volume of inbound calls by day of week and time of day, the reason for a call also provides us with information to

appropriately staff the telephones. The reason for the calls is important because you need to staff differently for the type of call, and you
need to work to reduce inbound call demand by anticipating patient
needs and enhancing call management. Staff can be asked to collect
this data for a one-week representative period. There will be errors
because it is difficult to collect the data during "a day in the life of
a medical practice"; however, this will provide good information to
help you optimally staff your telephones.

The graph of the inbound calls by reason for call for our sample
medical practice is provided in Exhibit 7.7. As demonstrated by this
graph, the highest call volume is for scheduling, followed by calls for
the nurse. The third highest call volume is for prescription renewals.

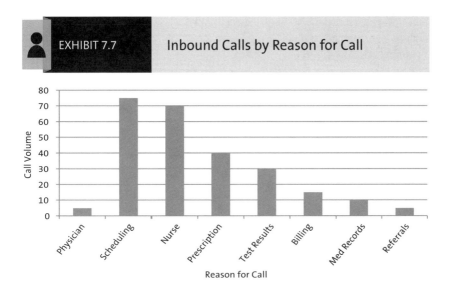

EXHIBIT 7.7   Inbound Calls by Reason for Call

These data provide additional information to develop the staffing
model for our sample medical practice. We now have an approxima-
tion of the volume of calls for nurse triage and the volume of calls
for appointment scheduling and other patient inquiries.

Identify the staff FTE required to manage the volume and type
of telephone calls — the inbound telephone demand — for your

medical practice. In our sample medical practice, we assume that medical practice leaders decided to have a nurse triage unit manage clinical calls and a patient scheduling unit manage administrative calls. We used the call data from our sample medical practice to build the required staffing FTE levels.

In Exhibit 7.8 we report the inbound telephone volume by day of the week that we computed earlier in this chapter. We then identify the type of inbound call by using the percentages that we obtained when we analyzed the reason for the inbound calls. In our sample medical practice we reflect clinical calls, scheduling calls, and all other calls (the latter is assumed to involve message-taking).

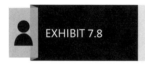

| EXHIBIT 7.8 | Inbound Calls by Day of Week and Reason for Call |

	Mon	Tue	Wed	Thu	Fri
Total inbound calls	250	200	150	100	50
Clinical calls (30% of total)	75	60	45	30	15
Scheduling (28% of total)	70	56	42	28	14
Messages (42% of total)	105	84	63	42	21

In order to build the staffing model for telephone management in our sample medical practice, we need to identify the expected staff workload ranges for telephone work. These were reported in Chapter 5, The Staff Workload Evaluation Process, and are restated in Exhibit 7.9.

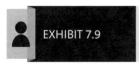

Work Function	Per Day	Per Hour
Telephones with messaging*	300–500	42–71
Telephones with routing (electronic system) only*	1,000–1,200	142–71
Appointment scheduling with no registration†	75–125	11–18
Appointment scheduling with full registration†	50–75	7–11
Telephone nurse triage*	65–85	8–12

*Source: Woodcock, Elizabeth W. 2009. *Mastering Patient Flow: Using Lean Thinking to Improve Your Practice Operations.* Englewood, Colo: Medical Group Management Association. Reprinted with permission.

†Source: Walker Keegan, Deborah; Elizabeth W. Woodcock; and Sara M. Larch. 2009. *The Physician Billing Process: 12 Potholes to Avoid in the Road to Getting Paid.* Englewood, Colo.: Medical Group Management Association. Reprinted with permission.

As we discussed in Chapter 5, it is important to make sure that the expected workload ranges are consistent with your particular medical practice. For purposes of this example for our sample medical practice, let's select the midpoint of each of the applicable expected staff workload ranges as follows:

Telephone nurse triage:	72 calls per day
Patient scheduling, no registration:	100 calls per day
Telephone messages (manual):	400 calls per day

To build the required staff FTEs, divide the call volume by the type of call by the expected workload to calculate the required staff FTEs to manage the type of call received by your medical practice. This calculation is demonstrated in Exhibit 7.10 for our sample medical practice. For example, on Monday there are 75 clinical calls. The expected workload range for telephone nurse triage in this practice is 72. Dividing 75 by 72, we calculate 1.04 staff FTE to manage the clinical call volume on Mondays. We continue this approach for each day of the week and each type of call.

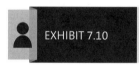

		Required Staff FTE to Manage Inbound Phones by Day of Week			
EXHIBIT 7.10					

	Mon	Tue	Wed	Thu	Fri
Total inbound calls	250	200	150	100	50
Clinical calls	75	60	45	30	15
Expected workload range	72	72	72	72	72
Total Required Clinical FTE	**1.04**	**.83**	**.63**	**.42**	**.21**
Scheduling	70	56	42	28	14
Expected workload range	100	100	100	100	100
Required staff FTE	*.70*	*.56*	*.42*	*.28*	*.14*
Messages	105	84	63	42	21
Expected workload range	400	400	400	400	400
Required staff FTE	*.26*	*.21*	*.16*	*.11*	*.05*
Total Required Schedule/ Message FTE	**.96**	**.77**	**.58**	**.39**	**.19**

Step 3: Redesign Work Processes

In step 3, determine the best work process for telephone management for clinical calls and nonclinical calls (such as appointment scheduling and messages) for your medical practice.

First, determine how you want to manage clinical calls. Options include:[2]

- Taking electronic or manual messages by telephone operators and routing to the nurse

- Connecting the caller to the nurse; if the nurse is not available, call goes to the nurse's voice mail and/or a message is taken

- Transferring caller to the voice mail at the nurse's desk, with the nurse checking voice mail throughout the day and responding to patients

- Using an automated message that instructs patients to leave a message and noting that the nurse will return the call at the end of the day

- Establishing a nurse telephone advice unit where nurses manage the inbound telephone calls in real time, with any overflow going to voice mail

- Other method

Next, determine your preferred work process for nonclinical calls. Options include:

- Using check-in and check-out staff to also manage inbound calls

- Having only one of the above — check-in or check-out — staff manage inbound calls

---

[2] URAC, a not-for-profit quality organization, recommends that clinical calls be answered in three rings, with a response provided to the patient within 30 minutes. A decision to be in line with these recommendations will obviously also affect the option you select for the management of inbound calls. See www.urac.org.

➤ Sending nonclinical calls to voice mail, with a staff member designated to transcribe the message and respond

➤ Establishing a separate staff scheduling/message unit to manage inbound calls

➤ Other method

The work process you select determines the staffing volume and skill mix of staff needed to manage telephones in your medical practice. It also impacts practice efficiency and the timeliness by which patients can access your medical practice. This decision also says volumes about whether your medical practice is a group practice where resources are shared among physicians or a collection of individual practices that are simply co-located, with limited resource sharing.

We recommend that the work of telephone management be separated from the work of the face-to-face visit with the patient. It is physically not possible for a single nurse to manage 25 to 30 patient visits per day and 100 to 120 inbound telephone calls per day and be effective in supporting the provider and the patient. Thus, we recommend the approach outlined in the fifth bullet above for the management of clinical calls. This involves the creation of a nurse telephone advice unit that manages calls in real time. This type of staffing model is facilitated by an electronic health record; however, this is not a requirement. Many medical practices have established a telephone nurse triage unit that works with clinical protocols and is able to manage the majority of calls without needing to request the medical record.

We recommend the fourth bullet above for the management of nonclinical calls. A formal telephone scheduling/message unit is designated to manage inbound calls, with staff focused on telephone responsibilities.

> We recommend that the work of telephone management be separated from the work of the face-to-face visit with the patient.

Further refine the staffing model by applying the same steps to the call data based on time of day. For example, you may find that inbound calls are highest in the morning, from 8:00 a.m. to 10:00 a.m., gradually declining until 1:00 p.m. when there is a second peak in call demand. Follow the same steps outlined earlier; however, refine the analysis by time of day in addition to day of week.

Step 4: Innovate Your Model

Determine the best work process for your medical practice and design a flexible staffing model around the type of work and quantity of work to be performed.

Based on this analysis, if there is no change to inbound call volume, our sample medical practice needs 1.00 FTE clinical support staff and 1.00 FTE telephone scheduler staff to manage the calls on Monday. On Tuesday and Wednesday these staff can be assigned a significant amount of other work to be performed during the course of the day, since a 1.00 FTE designation for each of the types of calls is not warranted based on the work. On Thursday and Friday a different staffing strategy can be used altogether. For example, one clinical support staff can be assigned to manage all of the inbound telephone volume (rather than a mix of scheduling and clinical staff); on Friday, in particular, this staff member should also be delegated significant other roles and responsibilities.

Take Action to Reduce Inbound Telephone Demand

Now that you know the reason for the inbound telephone calls to your practice, take action to reduce that demand. Exhibit 7.11 outlines some steps that you can take to reduce inbound telephone demand.[3] If you are successful in reducing the volume of inbound telephone calls, revisit your telephone staffing model, as it may be possible to reduce the number of staff devoted to telephone management and/or delegate additional responsibilities to these staff if their work volume declines.

---

[3] For a detailed discussion of these and other tools, see Woodcock, Elizabeth W. 2009. *Mastering Patient Flow: Using Lean Thinking to Improve Your Practice Operations, 3rd Edition.* Englewood, Colo.: Medical Group Management Association.

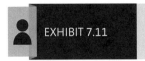

EXHIBIT 7.11   Actions to Reduce Telephone Demand

Type of Call	Action
Scheduling calls	Make sure templates extend out 12 months
	Make follow-up appointments at check-out
	Make postoperative appointments at the time of surgery scheduling
	Proactively manage care transitions; follow up with patients postdischarge and postemergency department visit
Test results	Set realistic expectations with patients
	Give patients a take-home tool that outlines how they will learn of their test results
	Create a closed-loop process to ensure the tests are administered, the results are received and reviewed, and patients are notified of results
	Give patients a top-five list of questions and answers specific to their visit, thereby anticipating patient needs and preventing a call
Prescription and medication	Place automated instruction to hang up and dial the pharmacy
	Ask patients if they need a renewal during their visit
	Create nursing clinical protocols
	Develop tools to recognize payer formularies
	If you need to reschedule patients, also check to see if you need to process a prescription renewal; some return appointments are scheduled to coincide with a renewal — for example, annual exams
General information	Forward callers to an automated line that details directions to the practice
	Direct patients to your medical practice's Website to obtain general information

INNOVATIVE STAFFING STRATEGIES FOR TELEPHONE MANAGEMENT

The most innovative process for telephone management is to replace the telephone with online patient access. Web portals through which patients schedule appointments, review their test results, and obtain prescription renewals, and secure messaging that enables patients to send text messages to their physician and care team are examples of innovative access channels that reduce inbound telephone demand.

> The most innovative process for telephone management is to replace the telephone with online patient access.

Even with these online solutions, most medical practices will still receive some telephone calls. Better-performing medical practices are able to manage these calls in one step by responding to the patient in real time. This is accomplished in the following ways:

> ➤ Separate patient flow work from telephone work

> ➤ Staff for the work

> ➤ Use electronic tools

Separate Patient Flow Work from Telephone Work

Assign staff to work either the internal patient flow process (the face-to-face visit) or the external patient flow process (the telephones), not both processes. This means that front office staff are deployed to manage either patient check-in/check-out OR the telephones, not both. This also means that clinical support staff are deployed to manage the patient flow process during the visit (visit preparation, retrieval, vital signs, rooming, assisting) OR the telephones, not both processes. In this fashion, the telephones can be managed in real time, reducing the need for message-taking and permitting more immediate feedback to patients in response to their needs.

Staff for the Work

Recognize the fluctuations in call volume by day of week, time of day, and reason for the call. Flexibly delegate the appropriate number of staff and skill mix of the staff consistent with the work.

Use Electronic Tools

Even if your medical practice does not use an electronic health record, implement electronic messages using standard templates. This permits messages to be routed to the appropriate party as needed and improves message clarity and timeliness. In addition, implement electronic appointment reminder systems to improve staff efficiency. Today's systems are more sophisticated than those of the past and can include reminders regarding materials for patients to bring to their appointments, and even remind them of outstanding account balances. Such systems can be further discriminated by having staff contact some of the patients by telephone outside of the automated queue, such as those with patient responsibility balances over a certain threshold or those who have a history of no-show or late arrival.

KEY QUESTIONS TO ADDRESS AS YOU STAFF THE TELEPHONES

- ➤ What is the volume of inbound calls by day of week and time of day?
- ➤ What is the workload of each staff member involved in telephone management?
- ➤ What are reasons for the inbound calls?
- ➤ Can sharing of telephone work occur (for example, can one nurse manage the inbound calls for three to five physicians)?
- ➤ What improvements to telephone management can be made to permit the call to be managed in one step involving real time call management?

➤ What steps can be taken to minimize inbound calls? For example, can electronic access methods for patients be expanded and/or can the medical practice better anticipate patients' inquiries, thereby preventing an inbound telephone call?

➤ What action can be taken to more effectively integrate telephone staff on the care team?

➤ Can we improve patient communication technology? For example, automate messages or use a Web portal to improve patient access?

SUMMARY

In this chapter, we built the staff FTE and skill mix required for telephone management by analyzing the work volume to be performed and the reason for inbound calls. We used expected staff workload ranges to build the staffing FTE and skill mix requirements based on day of the week and reason for the call. We then asked critical questions and explored staff role options in order to redesign the staffing model. In this fashion, you can innovate your staffing model and deploy the appropriate resources to effectively manage inbound telephone demand.

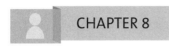
Staffing the Front Office: Patient Financial Clearance, Check-In, and Check-Out

The service encounter should be deliberately planned, carefully managed, and often [involve] rehearsed sets of behaviors.

—Service Encounters as Rites of Integration:
An Information-Processing Model

Your front office staff represent the first contact a patient has with your medical practice, and as such they serve not only as customer service representatives, but also as marketers and medical practice billers. This multifaceted role is challenging and requires a skill set that stretches between high interpersonal acumen and analytical skills. More and more, medical practices are recognizing that these staff are the key to patient access and satisfaction, as well as practice profitability.

In this chapter, we:

➤ Measure and analyze front office work

➤ Provide performance expectations regarding front office work

➤ Build a successful staffing model to manage patient check-in, check-out, and referral processes

➤ Share innovative staffing strategies for the front office

➤ Provide key questions to address as you staff the front office

KEY WORK FUNCTIONS FOR THE FRONT OFFICE

It is important that a medical practice address each work function of the front office as it relates to the what, who, how, and when this function is performed as part of its staffing deployment model. For the front office of a medical practice, key functions include:

➤ *Patient financial clearance.* Verify insurance and benefit eligibility, understand payment history, ensure authorizations are obtained prior to services performed.

➤ *Patient check-in.* Verify information, obtain and post time-of-service payments, obtain waivers and patient signatures — for example, Health Insurance Portability and Accountability Act (HIPAA) notification.

➤ *Patient check-out.* Schedule patient follow-up appointments, schedule procedures, process outbound referrals, enter outpatient charges, and work pre-adjudication claim edits.

The detailed work involved in each of these work functions is described in the following sections.

Patient Financial Clearance/Previsit Process

One of the key role changes in the consumer-directed healthcare environment is that of patient financial clearance. Patient financial clearance involves all of the steps necessary for the business of medicine to be accurately conducted. This work is now typically conducted prior to patients arriving for their scheduled visits and includes insurance verification, eligibility verification, demographic verification, point-of-care payment determination, and referral and authorization verification.

Patient Check-In Process

Patient check-in involves the following tasks:

- ➤ Verifying patient demographic and insurance information
- ➤ Collecting time-of-service payments and issuing receipts
- ➤ Obtaining waiver signatures
- ➤ Scanning insurance cards for new patients, patients with an insurance change, and patients who received new cards from their carrier (even if not an insurance change), and reviewing and verifying insurance cards with system information (note that this step is not needed if formal insurance verification has been performed at previsit unless concerns regarding patient identity are an issue)

Medical records are maintained in the back office area (creating a paperless front office). All updates from a business standpoint are made in real time online via the practice management system. Announcement of patient arrival to the physician and clinical support staff typically occurs online and/or via printing of charge tickets and/or labels in the back office area. Cash balancing is conducted at the end of the day, with appropriate internal controls and security of cash, checks, and credit and debit cards. Assurance is made that HIPAA privacy forms are signed and recorded in the system. The check-in staff may schedule the next appointment at check-in (for example, well-child exam or follow-up chemotherapy treatment), anticipating the follow-up appointment that is needed for a particular type of patient.

> The front office staff largely determine whether or not a clean claim is submitted to payers.

Patient Check-Out Process

Check-out staff schedule follow-up appointments and appointments for imaging, laboratory, and other procedures. The reason for the visit is placed into the practice management system to serve as a queue for the clinical previsit preparation required for the next appointment. The check-out staff also conduct referral processing and perform charge entry for outpatient activity.

Patients present at check-out with an order sheet that includes a patient label and instructions for the next appointment, test, or procedures, or staff go online to view the electronic note to determine next steps. Patient may also present with his or her charge ticket; however, in many medical practices, the charge ticket is maintained in the back office area, or the charge is electronically entered and no hard copy charge ticket is produced.

PERFORMANCE EXPECTATIONS FOR THE FRONT OFFICE STAFF

The skills needed for a service encounter include interpersonal acumen, communication skills, customer sensitivity, decisiveness, energy, flexibility, follow-up, impact, initiative, integrity, job knowledge, judgment, motivation to serve, persuasiveness, planning, resilience, situation analysis, and work standards.[1] Add to that the requirements of today's medical practice — knowledge of payer requirements, how to determine patient responsibility payments, when to obtain authorizations, how to determine coordination of benefits, charge entry, and other similar "business-of-medicine" issues that are highly complex — and it is clear that the front office staff play the role of marketer, biller, information processor, reimbursement manager, and a host of other roles. Today's front office is sophisticated and requires sophisticated members on the care team.

---

[1] Bernthal, Paul, and James Davis. Monograph. *Service Skills in the Workplace*. Development Dimensions International, Inc. Revised MMIV, pp. 1–28. List found on p. 6. www.ddiworld.com. Accessed 11/09/10.

Consistent with that sophistication, we expect a level of performance and contribution from these staff far greater than in the past. Exhibit 8.1 outlines the work quantity expected of the front office staff (note that this was first presented in Chapter 5, The Staff Workload Evaluation Process, and is restated here).

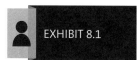

EXHIBIT 8.1 — Expected Staff Workload Ranges for Front Office

Work Function	Per Day	Per Hour
Registration with insurance verification (on-site or previsit)	60–80	9–11
Patient check-in with registration verification only	100–130	14–19
Patient check-in with registration verification and cashiering only	75–100	11–14
Check-out with scheduling and cashiering	70–90	10–13
Check-out with scheduling, cashiering, and charge entry	60–80	9–11
Referrals (inbound or outbound)	70–90	10–13

Source: Walker Keegan, Deborah L.; Elizabeth W. Woodcock; and Sara M. Larch. 2009. *The Physician Billing Process: 12 Potholes to Avoid in the Road to Getting Paid*. Englewood, Colo.: Medical Group Management Association. Reprinted with permission.

In addition to work quantity, we expect a high level of quality in the work. The front office staff largely determine whether or not a clean claim is submitted to payers. They are responsible for securing and verifying patient demographic and insurance information, as well as obtaining payment at the point of care. Quality expectations for their work include the following:

- ⇒ Patient Financial Clearance
  - Registration errors are less than 2 percent of claim edits and claim denials[2]
  - All authorizations are obtained prior to the visit
  - The medical practice knows the amount to be collected at the point of care for each patient

- ⇒ Patient Check-In
  - Patients are not asked to repeat information that has already been provided
  - Scanning of insurance cards takes place at each visit (or at established policy levels)
  - Copayments are collected 98 percent of the time[3]
  - Co-insurance, deductibles, and patient responsibility balances are collected 75 percent of the time[4]
  - An electronic receipt is provided to the patient for each payment received

- ⇒ Patient Check-Out
  - Follow-up appointments include the reasons for the follow-up visits
  - Patients are provided with information and tools so they know next steps and do not have to "go fish" for information after their visit
  - Procedures and tests are scheduled consistent with physician orders
  - Referral processes are completed to permit transition of patient to specialist or to procedure

---

[2] Walker Keegan, Deborah L.; Elizabeth W. Woodcock; and Sara M. Larch. 2009. *The Physician Billing Process: 12 Potholes to Avoid in the Road to Getting Paid.* Englewood, Colo.: Medical Group Management Association.

[3] Ibid.

[4] Ibid.

- Charge entry is accurate, with claim edits due to charge entry errors less than 2 percent of charges entered[5]
- Charges are entered the same day as they are received
- Pre-adjudication claim edits are worked the same day as they are received

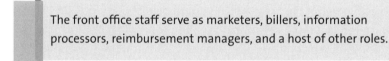

The front office staff serve as marketers, billers, information processors, reimbursement managers, and a host of other roles.

BUILD THE FRONT OFFICE STAFFING MODEL

To build the staffing model for front office work, proceed through the four-step process to optimal staffing first outlined in Chapter 3:

1. *Benchmark staff full-time equivalents (FTEs) and costs*

   Benchmark the staff involved in the front office. The MGMA Cost Survey staff category of "total front office staff" and its work function level of "medical receptionists" typically are used for this benchmarking analysis.

2. *Evaluate staff workload*

   The patient visit volume is the unit of work for patient check-in and patient check-out staff. The number of referrals to be processed is the unit of work for referral management staff.

   Collect a representative work sample. Determine the patient visit volume for a one-week period by day of week and session per day. Do not select a peak volume period for this sample. The goal is to staff for the typical work volume and then use other techniques to manage peak volume demand.

   Build the staff based on the expected workload ranges. Use the expected staff workload process we described in

---

[5] Ibid.

Chapter 5 to build the number of staff required for the work quantity. First, evaluate the expected staff workload ranges (in Exhibit 8.1) to determine if they are consistent with your medical practice, then measure the work volume of your staff and analyze the performance gaps.

An example of that approach is provided in Exhibit 8.2 for our sample medical practice. In this exhibit, a range of 1.27 to 3.04 FTE staff are required to manage the morning clinic session and .25 to 3.56 FTEs are required to manage the afternoon clinic session, depending on the day of the week. Note the wide variability by day of week and session per day. A further differentiation based on hours within each session can also be computed.

Consistent with one of the themes of this book, a medical practice needs to staff for the work. Therefore, if this medical practice is not able to reduce the patient visit variation, its staffing deployment model needs to be flexible based on day of week and session per day consistent with the work. If a flexible model is not adopted, then the medical practice will not be staffed at optimal levels. On various sessions per day it will have either more or fewer staff needed to conduct the work.

For medical practices with referral management activity, the unit of work is the number of referrals to be processed. Exhibit 8.2 outlines the expectation related to work quantity for referral management staff. We typically expect referral processors to manage 70 to 90 inbound and/or outbound referrals per day or 10 to 13 per hour. The work of referral management typically includes contact with payers and/or patients, processing the required paperwork, securing (and following up to obtain) approval, scheduling appointments, and submitting the appropriate authorizations.

3. *Redesign work processes*

Determine the work to be performed by the front office staff. For example, a decision could be made to eliminate the check-in station, with data verification and time-of-service payments collected by the medical assistant when

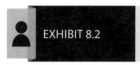

EXHIBIT 8.2	Staffing for Patient Check-In and Check-Out (Including Charge Entry)				
	Mon	**Tue**	**Wed**	**Thu**	**Fri**
Morning Clinic Visits	50	45	40	60	25
FTE required for check-in	1.11	1.00	.89	1.33	.56
FTE required for check-out	1.43	1.29	1.14	1.71	.71
Total FTE Required AM	**2.54**	**2.29**	**2.03**	**3.04**	**1.27**
Afternoon Clinic Visits	70	50	45	55	5
FTE required for check-in	1.56	1.11	1.00	1.22	.11
FTE required for check-out	2.00	1.43	1.29	1.57	.14
Total FTE Required PM	**3.56**	**2.54**	**2.29**	**2.79**	**.25**

Notes: Staff workload expectation for patient check-in and cashiering: 75 to 100 per day; 90 used in above table (45 each half-day clinic session).

Staff workload expectation for patient check-out, scheduling, and charge entry: 60 to 80 per day; 70 used in above table (35 each half-day clinic session).

the patient is in the exam room. A decision at this step needs to be made regarding the full work scope to be delegated to front office staff.

Equally important is the decision as to "who" should perform the work. Two examples are provided to help redesign the work processes of front office staff.

Example 1: Patient Financial Clearance. Exhibit 8.3 outlines three separate groups of staff that can be involved in this work function — scheduling staff, front office staff, and billing staff. In addition, two work options within each of these categories are listed. Any one of these staffing models will work, and as part of the work redesign step, the specific process and the identification of the staff to be involved in the process need to be determined.

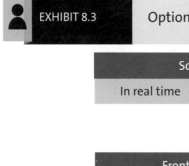

EXHIBIT 8.3   Options for Patient Financial Clearance

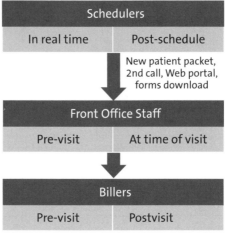

Schedulers	
In real time	Post-schedule

New patient packet,
2nd call, Web portal,
forms download

Front Office Staff	
Pre-visit	At time of visit

Billers	
Pre-visit	Postvisit

Example 2: Procedure Scheduling. Procedure scheduling can be conducted in the traditional model — by having the patient walk to the check-out or scheduling desk — by having the patient walk to the nurses' station, by having a scheduler travel to the patient in the exam room, by having a clinical support staff member manage this process at the completion of the exam while the patient is in the exam room, or by sending the patient home and calling the patient at a subsequent time. Any of these options can be designed to work (though having the staff travel to the patient rather than the other way around is optimal), but the important point is to determine the work process and the type of staff to be involved in that process for your medical practice.

4. *Innovate your model*

Innovate your front office staffing model consistent with the work and the redesigned work processes.

INNOVATIVE STAFFING STRATEGIES FOR THE FRONT OFFICE

With electronic health records and today's practice management systems, there is no need to continue to manage the patient check-in and check-out processes in the traditional in-person, sequential pattern. Innovative staffing strategies for the front desk are now presented.[6]

> Eliminate waiting and queuing and bring the work to the patient. Consider eliminating the check-in and check-out desks and conduct this work in the exam room.

Patient Financial Clearance

> *Online registration.* Conduct online patient preregistration; ask patients to enter information or update information online and/or print out registration forms that they can bring with them to the appointment, thereby delegating this work to the patient.

> *Automated insurance verification.* Automate the insurance verification process for your medical practice. Many medical practices have contracted with vendors to automate this function, with staff then focused on obtaining updated information for patient outliers who do not pass this verification screening.

> *Previsit payment reminders.* Contact patients by telephone to obtain outstanding patient responsibility payments (by credit or debit card) before they present for appointments, thereby minimizing this work at the front desk and ensuring payment.

---

[6] For more front desk strategies, see Woodcock, Elizabeth W. 2011. *Front Office Success: How to Satisfy Patients and Boost the Bottom Line.* Englewood, Colo.: Medical Group Management Association.

Patient Check-In

> *Eliminate the queue.* Eliminate waiting and queuing and bring the work to the patient. Immediately room the patient at time of presentation and collect any time-of-service payments while the patient is in the exam room.

> *Flexible staffing model.* Do not staff for peak periods. Create notification/alert systems (like a grocery store when a line at the check-out area begins to form).

> *Patient self check-in.* Implement kiosks for patient check-in, thereby delegating work to the patient, who can perform this function electronically at your medical practice.

> *Stagger start times.* By staggering visit times for physicians, the staff can attend to the full scope of work for each patient, which is often difficult to accomplish with large numbers of patients arriving at the same time for appointments.

Patient Check-Out

> *Eliminate the queue.* Eliminate waiting and queuing and bring the work to the patient. Ask clinical staff to schedule follow-up appointments and procedures while the patient is in the exam room or have schedulers travel to the exam room to interact with patients and eliminate the check-out desk.

> *Co-locate staff.* Co-locate check-in and check-out staff and cross-train them so they can assist each other during peak periods. For example, if the first patient is scheduled at 8:00 a.m., there will not be any patients to check out until approximately 8:30 a.m. Staff can be assigned to help with check-in during that 30-minute period. Push back the chairs and have all staff stand during this time so they can be optimally effective in these dual roles.

> *Collect patient payments prior to elective service.* Collect patient payment for upcoming elective procedures and services prior to the procedure being performed (if your contracts permit).

Be a financial advocate for patients and help them understand what their insurance will pay and what their insurance indicates is their responsibility — and ensure that your practice is paid in a timely fashion.

➤ *Do not batch work.* Enter charges throughout the day rather than wait until day-end. Waiting is a form of batching and delaying the work.[7]

➤ *Identify additional work functions.* Identify forms that can be partially completed by front office staff during downtime and other similar episodic work functions.

➤ *Centralize referral processing.* Centralize referral processing with one or two staff, rather than each staff member conducting this function. This creates efficiencies in the work performed and frees up staff to attend to other important work functions.

KEY QUESTIONS TO ADDRESS AS YOU STAFF THE FRONT OFFICE

➤ What steps can be taken to prepare business functions in advance of the visit?

➤ Can steps be taken to reduce variable work levels for the staff? Can visit times be staggered or lagged to reduce work variation?

➤ Is there work that patients can conduct online that will streamline their visit experience?

➤ Can work steps be combined rather than involve process handoffs between staff?

➤ Can work accuracy be improved by employing a different staffing model?

➤ Is there an opportunity to centralize work functions such as referral management?

➤ Can work processes become more efficient through automation?

---

[7] Woodcock, Elizabeth W. 2009. *Mastering Patient Flow: Using Lean Thinking to Improve Your Practice Operations.* Englewood, Colo.: Medical Group Management Association.

SUMMARY

In today's medical practices, there are fewer and fewer human touches with the patient. Patients can access information and appointments via the medical practice's Web portal, and they may receive virtual medicine through secure messaging in between their annual face-to-face visits with the physician. With fewer human touches, we need to make sure that the ones patients do have matter. Your front office staff are the visible representation of your medical practice. Their work is critical, not only for financial viability, but also for patient access and service delivery.

In this chapter, we described the key work functions of front office staff, how to build a successful staffing deployment model for the front office, and innovative staffing strategies that can take your medical practice to the next level of performance.

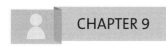

CHAPTER 9

Staffing the Visit: Clinical Support Staff

When I visit a medical practice and the nurses are sitting in pods and are on the phone, I typically know what I will see: The physician will be doing more and more of the work himself.

—Deborah Walker Keegan, PhD, FACMPE

The clinical support staff are those care team members who interact with the physician and patient to deliver patient care. Determining the right combination of registered nurses (RNs), licensed practical nurses (LPNs), and medical assistants (MAs) for the work and delegating appropriate work are critical if we are to optimize their contribution to the care team.

In this chapter, we:

⇾ Measure and analyze the work of clinical support staff

⇾ Provide performance expectations for clinical support staff

⇾ Build a successful staffing model in support of the provider and patient visit

⇾ Share innovative staffing strategies for patient visit support

⇾ Provide key questions to address as you staff for the visit

WORK FUNCTIONS FOR CLINICAL SUPPORT STAFF

Clinical support staff are typically deployed to support the patient visit (the internal patient flow process), respond to patients' calls requiring triage and advice (the external patient flow process), and manage secure online messages with patients related to their care (the virtual patient flow process). Each of these work functions is further described in the following sections.

Clinical Support Staff and the Patient Visit

Clinical staff who support the patient visit and patient flow should anticipate both physician and patient needs and actively participate in the patient visit itself. We expect to see these staff up on their feet in support of patient flow in the medical practice. Work functions delegated to these staff include:

> ➤ *Previsit clinical preparation.* Anticipate patient, visit, exam room, and procedure needs; identify outstanding clinical needs of patients (for example, via disease registries).

> ➤ *Patient flow support.* Retrieve patient, take vital signs, obtain medication history, obtain reason for visit, prepare patient for the exam, and keep the provider on time.

> ➤ *Procedure support.* Anticipate needs of physician and patient for procedures, participate in procedures, administer immunizations, and conduct nursing visits, such as blood pressure checks, allergy shots, complex wound care management, and other similar nursing tasks.

> ➤ *Patient discharge support.* Educate patients, discharge patients from the exam room, schedule and/or arrange for follow-up procedures and tests, and review charge ticket for completion.

Clinical staff who support the patient visit and patient flow should be up on their feet anticipating both physician and patient needs and actively participating in the actual patient visit.

Clinical Support Staff and Nurse Triage

The most efficient organization of nurse triage and advice staff is to co-locate these staff to permit resource sharing and knowledge support. Their key work functions include:

➤ *Telephone advice/triage.* Respond to patient inquiries, following clinical guidelines and protocols consistent with licensure (such as prescription renewal and medication questions).

➤ *Laboratory and test results.* Manage a closed-loop system to ensure all tests are administered, results are received and reviewed, alert physician to abnormal results, and ensure systematic communication with patients regarding results and next steps.

CLINICAL STAFF SKILL MIX

What is the best mix of clinical support staff involving RNs, LPNs, and MAs in a medical practice? The answer to that question is: It depends. It depends on a host of issues, including:

➤ Role delegation by the physician

➤ The specialty of the medical practice's physicians

➤ The type of patients presenting to the medical practice

➤ The licensure requirements of the particular state as it relates to delegated authority

➤ The local job market and the availability of specific clinical support staff types

Thus, there is no one right answer as to best skill mix for all medical practices. Consistent with the themes in this book, we need to staff for the work. The licensure that is needed is wholly dependent on the work that has been delegated to the clinical support staff. What we strive to do is match the work with the appropriate level of staff needed to perform the work. In addition, we seek to use licensed staff wisely. That is, simply assigning a full-time nurse to each physician to manage the occasional clinical question or the occasional required visit support can be replaced with a staffing model that focuses the work requiring licensed staff.

BENCHMARKING CLINICAL STAFF

To determine whether you have the correct number and skill mix of clinical staff, first benchmark these staff to the available survey instruments. In this fashion, a medical practice can determine if it has a skill mix consistent with peer practices in the same specialty. As outlined in Chapter 4, The Staff Benchmarking Process, benchmarks are available not only at the level of RN, LPN, and MA, but also at the categorical level of total clinical support staff (which combines each of the three functions). This will allow you to compare your overall clinical staffing support (regardless of skill mix of these staff) and view the skill mix of RNs, LPNs, and MAs that are used in other medical practices to determine whether there is an opportunity related to the volume of clinical support staff and the skill mix of these staff in your medical practice.

Experts estimate that up to 75 percent of what the nurse does is repeated by the physician. If that is the case in your medical practice, decide who should perform the work rather than perpetuate this rework. If the physician insists on doing the work, then you may not need an LPN, for example; a change in skill mix to a MA may be more appropriate.

> The most efficient organization of nurse triage and advice staff is to co-locate these staff to permit resource sharing and knowledge support.

PERFORMANCE EXPECTATIONS FOR CLINICAL SUPPORT STAFF

Develop specific performance expectations for clinical staff and institute competency assessments to ensure that the staff are performing high-quality work.

In terms of work quantity, the unit of work for the clinical support staff varies based on their work delegation as follows:

➤ *Patient flow support.* The unit of work is the patient visit volume and type.

➤ *Telephone nurse triage.* The unit of work is the inbound telephone call volume.

➤ *Virtual medicine.* The unit of work is the number of secure message threads and/or the number of patients for which care and case management is to occur.

The expected workload range for clinical support staff is reported in Exhibit 9.1. Note that these ranges are generally broad, because the specific type of patient and specific clinical intervention will dictate the amount of time required for the clinical staff.

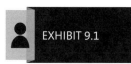 **EXHIBIT 9.1** **Expected Staff Workload Ranges for Clinical Support**

Work Function	Per Day	Per Hour
Telephone nurse triage*	65–85	8–12
Patient intake: Patient rooming, vital signs	Variable based on work that can be delegated; typically, 25 to 40 patients per day	N/A
Visit support: Nurse visit support, procedures, education	Variable based on work that can be delegated; typically, 25 to 40 patients per day	N/A
Health and wellness coaching	Variable, based on type of coaching provided; see Chapter 12: Staffing the Medical Home Model for a detailed discussion	N/A

N/A = not applicable

Note: The expected staff workload range assumes full nurse triage and advice, not simply prescription renewals or responding to inquiries of a nonclinical nature, such as scheduling or information requests.

*Source: Woodcock, Elizabeth W. 2009. *Mastering Patient Flow: Using Lean Thinking to Improve Your Practice Operations.* Englewood, Colo.: Medical Group Management Association. Reprinted with permission.

BUILD A CLINICAL STAFF SUPPORT MODEL

Follow the four-step model to optimal staffing to develop a successful clinical staff support model:

1. *Benchmark staff full-time equivalents (FTEs) and costs*
    Benchmark the clinical support staff following the steps described in Chapter 4. The categorical level of these staff is "total clinical support staff" reported in the MGMA Cost Survey instrument. Benchmarking at this and the functional levels of RN, LPN, and MA helps to identify whether you have more or fewer clinical support staff than peer practices and whether your skill mix of these staff is consistent with benchmark norms.

2. *Evaluate staff workload*
    The unit of work for clinical support staff varies based on the work they are tasked to perform. For staff involved in patient flow support, the unit of work is the volume of patient visits and the type of support provided for the visit. For staff involved in telephones, the unit of work is the volume of telephone calls requiring nurse triage and advice. For clinical staff serving as case managers and health and wellness coaches, the number of cases assigned to the staff is the unit of work. Finally, for clinical staff involved in online support to the patient, the unit of work is the volume of secure message threads to be managed. Identify the number of patient visits and number of inbound telephone calls and secure messages that need to be managed during a representative one-week period. Identify these workloads based on day of week and session per day. Follow the expected staff workload evaluation process. As we outlined in Chapter 5, build the staffing levels that are needed consistent with the work type and work volume.

    Compare this built clinical staff model with your current model and perform a gap analysis, asking and answering critical questions regarding your model.

3. *Redesign work processes*

   Determine the scope of work to be performed by the clinical staff. For example, what rooming and vital signs are expected? What level of autonomy does the nurse have in responding to patient telephone inquiries? What role are the staff expected to play in support of the physician and the patient? This will assist in identifying the approximate time required by the clinical staff to perform their work functions as well as the specific licensure needed for the work.

4. *Innovate your model*

   Build the staff based on the expected staff workload ranges and type of work delegated to the staff and innovate your model.

Let's look at some samples of problematic clinical support models and the questions that should be asked and answered of these models as the medical practice works to improve staffing for the patient visit.

Example 1: A Whole Lot of Nurses

This pediatric practice has five physicians. Each physician is assigned his or her 1.00 FTE LPN, and there is also a 1.00 FTE RN who administers allergy shots. To determine if this model is appropriate, these questions need to be addressed:

- Does each physician work 10 sessions per week?
- How many patients do the physicians see?
- What type of work do the LPNs perform?
- Do the LPNs manage both the patient flow process and the telephone process?
- Are LPNs required for each of the work functions performed?
- Are LPNs performing any nursing visits?
- How many allergy shots are administered by the RN?

➤ What is the distribution of allergy shots by day of week and time of day?

➤ What work functions could be delegated to a medical assistant or other staff member?

Example 2: Dr. Green on the Phone

Dr. Green is routinely interrupted to respond to telephone inquiries. Analysis of the time spent handling telephone calls is 10 minutes each hour (80 minutes per day). Can a change to the clinical support model improve the physician's efficiency and productivity? Ask and answer the following questions:

➤ What types of telephone calls are received?

➤ What is the turnaround time required for these calls?

➤ Can an LPN manage some or all of the calls?

➤ What are the nurses doing in the medical practice? Can they assume the role of telephone management for these calls?

➤ What is the opportunity cost of the physician to manage the telephone calls? For example, is the physician seeing lower patient visit volumes due to his telephone responsibilities? What is the cost per visit of the physician's time?

By identifying your current clinical staffing deployment model, performing a gap analysis regarding work quantity, and asking and answering key questions regarding your model, you can identify opportunities for improvement to the clinical staffing model for your practice.

INNOVATIVE STAFFING STRATEGIES FOR CLINICAL SUPPORT

Evaluate the following innovative strategies for deploying clinical support staff in your medical practice.

Group Practice Orientation

As you build your staffing model for the visit, determine whether the physicians can move to more of a group practice approach to care. That is, instead of each physician being assigned one medical assistant or nurse who does everything in support of the patient visit and the telephones, determine if a shared resource can be allocated. For example, one telephone nurse can support three to six physicians (depending on the type of practice and the inbound call volume and type of call). As another example, if physicians are not working 10 sessions per week in the clinic, determine if their clinical support staff can be deployed to assist other physicians and/or be flexibly scheduled not to work. As a final example, consider assigning medical assistants to manage patient flow, a shared RN or LPN to manage the phones, and a shared RN or LPN to assist with procedures, injections, wound care, and other similar nursing duties. In this fashion, you are linking resources in support of the work, not simply assigning clinical support staff to a physician on a permanent basis regardless of the workload or type of work.

Regardless of whether a group practice approach is emphasized by your medical practice, it is not physically possible for a single nurse to provide patient flow and visit support for 25 to 30 patients and also manage 100 to 120 calls in a timely and accurate fashion. Identify clinical staff to manage patient flow and visit support and separate clinical staff to manage telephone calls and virtual medicine. In this fashion, the staff can be fully devoted to these roles rather than attempting to manage both processes simultaneously.

> It is not physically possible for a single nurse to provide patient flow and visit support for 25 to 30 patient visits and also manage 100 to 120 calls in a timely and accurate fashion. Identify clinical staff to manage patient flow and visit support and separate clinical staff to manage telephone calls and virtual medicine.

Nursing Scope

The traditional nursing roles in the medical practice are expanding. New roles for licensed nurses include care and case management, guided care, and other patient outreach and coaching activities to assist patients. In Chapter 12, Staffing the Medical Home Model, a host of additional roles for nursing staff is outlined and should be considered for today's care team. Beyond these new roles, to meet the meaningful use criteria established for incentive payments for electronic health records, enhanced team engagement in the patient visit is needed. The changing staff roles due to electronic health records are discussed in Chapter 11.

Nurse–Physician Leverage Model

In a nurse–physician visit model, the nurse takes the social and medical history from the patient and presents the patient to the physician in front of the patient. This is similar to a resident presenting the patient to an attending physician. In this innovative model, the nurse spends significant time with the patient to garner the patient's history and current problems, with the physician focused on the exam and treatment plan, followed by the nurse providing education and patient support. Both the nurse and physician are actively involved in the patient visit; after the nurse's work-up of the patient, the work is performed in a synchronous fashion.[1]

Staffing the Exam Rooms

For highly productive medical practices, consider staffing the exam rooms. Each medical assistant (or other clinical support staff, depending on work delegation) is assigned a specific exam room. His or her job is to room the patient, assist with the visit — including assisting with the exam and functioning as a scribe for the physi-

---

[1] The recognized author of this model for family medicine is Dr. Peter Anderson. More information can be found at www.familyteamcare.org and Anderson, Peter, and Marc D. Halley. 2008 "A new approach to making your doctor–nurse team more productive." *Fam Pract Manag.* 15(17):35–40.

cian — and discharging the patient from the exam room. Repeat this process throughout the day. We typically recommend this model for busy dermatology and ophthalmology practices, in particular; however, other specialties can also benefit from this staffing deployment model.

Central Treatment Area

Another model that is used in highly productive practices is to centralize a treatment area in the suite where managing wound care, removing sutures, taking blood pressure, administering injections and immunizations, and other similar nursing functions that typically require licensure takes place. By centralizing these services, the nursing care provided to patients can take place outside of the physician's assigned exam room, with dedicated staff devoted to these functions. If a central treatment area is developed, it is important to ensure nonduplication of nursing staff, since much of their work is consolidated into this central treatment area, rather than in the exam rooms. Key roles and responsibilities for staff assigned to a central treatment area include:

➢ Nursing support for procedures and wound care

➢ Nursing support for injections and immunizations

➢ Nursing support for scheduled nursing visits, for example, blood pressure checks

Nurse Advice Unit

A nurse advice unit to manage inbound and outbound call volume is an efficient staffing model for telephone management — and it reduces the time to respond to patient telephone inquiries, since staff are fully devoted to this function. Some medical practices rotate the patient flow nurse and the telephone nurse each week to ensure that each is cross-trained and has work variety.

Key roles and responsibilities for nurses assigned to triage and advice include:

- Respond to inbound clinical telephone calls and perform nurse triage and advice
- Place outbound calls as directed by physician, for example, lab results and medication changes, and provide follow-up instruction to patients
- Manage and work patient logs, for example, mammography, Pap smears, and anticoagulation logs

Care Team Nurse

Another innovative model is to identify a team nurse to perform complex patient coordination and nursing visits (such as first obstetrical visit, diabetic education, and complex wound care) and to educate and counsel patients.

Key roles and responsibilities for a care team nurse include:

- Coordinate care delivery for complex patients
- Follow high-risk patients
- Preview appointment schedules and identify patient issues pertinent to the patient visit
- Manage handoffs to other caregivers, for example, home health
- Perform nursing visits
- Assist with procedures

Virtual Medicine Support

More medical practices today are involving clinical staff in virtual medicine, including managing secure message threads and the Web portal. In these situations, the clinical staff use established clinical protocols to provide advice and support to patients and respond to patient inquiries. In a number of medical practices, the secure message volume from patients is increasing, reducing face-to-face visits and also reducing inbound telephone call volume from patients. We expect to see this area expand significantly as changes to healthcare reimbursement are introduced to recognize expanded patient access models of care and accountable care.

Enhanced Communication Methods

Physician and Clinical Support Staff

More and more medical practices are utilizing technology to enhance communication between the physician and the clinical support staff. This permits the physician to stay in the exam room to complete the exam rather than leave the exam room to look for the nurse. If electronic communication methods such as wireless communication and text messages are not instituted, simple methods to improve communication and permit synchronous work by physicians and clinical support staff such as the following can be used:

- *Discharge flow sheet.* A discharge flow sheet is left in the door to alert the nurse to nursing support or needed follow-up.

- *Flags or light systems.* A flag or light is used to signal the need for clinical support staff and/or next steps for the patient in the patient flow process, for example, need for imaging or EKG.

These methods improve the efficiency of both the physician and the clinical support staff. Without improving communication to permit synchronous work, it is likely that higher levels of clinical support staff are required — or lower levels of physician productivity ensue — due to queuing and waiting built into the work flow.

Medical Practice and Patient

Communication between the medical practice and the patient should not always involve the patient placing a telephone call to the practice to ask for the nurse. Patient needs should be anticipated and information should be provided to patients so they do not have to personally call the medical practice for each and every issue. This, too, improves the efficiency by which the clinical staff conduct their work. Consider the following tools to prevent the call:

➤ *Formal reporting process.* Adopt a systematic process to review lab and test results and report results to patients. A closed-loop lab/test system ensures that tests are performed, results are received and reviewed, and results are communicated to the patient.

➤ *Visit summary take-home.* Provide a visit summary sheet to patients so that they know their diagnosis and current and next steps related to their treatment plan. This summary sheet also informs patients when and how to expect their test results (note that a visit summary is one of the core criteria for meaningful use of the electronic health record as part of the government's incentive program).

KEY QUESTIONS TO ADDRESS AS YOU STAFF THE VISIT

➤ What work functions have been delegated to each clinical support staff?

➤ How does the clinical support staff volume compare with available benchmarks in similar practices? What is the skill mix of the benchmarks in comparison to the medical practice?

➤ What steps are taken to prepare for the visit (for example, chart prep, exam room prep, patient prep, procedure prep)? Is additional visit preparation needed?

➤ How are patient telephone calls related to clinical issues managed? What are the reasons for the calls and what is the current turnaround time to get back with the patient?

➤ What work functions are licensed clinical support staff doing that could be delegated to nonlicensed staff?

➤ Can sharing of staff in a group practice model improve work scope and focus the clinical staff on discrete work functions?

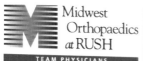

TEAM PHYSICIANS
Chicago White Sox & Chicago Bulls

Mary F. Rodts,
DNP, CNP, ONC, FAAN
Nurse Practitioner
Chief Operating Officer

1611 West Harrison Street, Suite 300
Chicago, Illinois 60612
P 312.432.2445 • F 708.492.5445

mrodts@rushortho.com

www.rushortho.com

➤ Are there other staffing deployment models that will better meet physician and/or patient needs?

➤ What communication channels can be developed to improve provider-nurse and practice-patient communication?

SUMMARY

In this chapter, we discussed how to analyze and build a clinical staff model for your medical practice. We also shared innovative models used in many of today's medical practices. By separating the patient flow nursing support from the phone and virtual nursing support, we can support the physician and the patient as part of a well-coordinated care team, with full delegation of resources to these important patient flow processes.

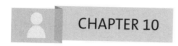

CHAPTER 10

Staffing the Billing Office[1]

The key to an effective revenue cycle is to avoid "potholes" in the road to getting paid. By deploying the right staff doing the right things you can optimize revenue performance for your practice.

— The Physician Billing Process: 12 Potholes
to Avoid in the Road to Getting Paid

At some point we expect to have innovations in physician billing. Picture a new model where the patient swipes a card at check-out and data are directly submitted from your electronic health record to the payer, with the payer immediately transferring money to your bank account. When that time comes, it will truly revolutionize the staffing strategy used for billing and collection work.

We certainly do not have that instantaneous reimbursement model in place today. You are instead faced with a convoluted and complex revenue cycle that you need to maneuver to get reimbursed for the services you provide in your medical practice. This requires a formal structuring of the work processes and

---

[1] This chapter is based on the book, *The Physician Billing Process: 12 Potholes to Avoid in the Road to Getting Paid* by Deborah Walker Keegan, Elizabeth W. Woodcock, and Sara M. Larch (Medical Group Management Association, 2009). Portions of the book are restated in this chapter and reprinted with permission.

handoffs among physicians and staff involved in both front-end and back-end billing functions.

In this chapter, we:

➤ Present billing office work functions

➤ Build a successful staffing model to manage back-end billing

➤ Provide performance expectations for billing and collections

➤ Share innovative staffing strategies for the billing office

➤ Provide questions to address as you staff your billing office

BILLING OFFICE WORK FUNCTIONS

The work involved in billing and collections is typically divided into front-end billing and back-end billing functions.

Work Functions for Front-End Billing

Front-end billing functions include the following key areas: credentialing, registration and scheduling, patient financial clearance, patient check-in and check-out, coding, charge capture, charge entry, and collection of time-of-service payments. In Chapter 8, Staffing the Front Office, we discussed the work functions related to patient financial clearance, patient check-in, and patient check-out, and how to build a successful staffing model for this work.

Work Functions for Back-End Billing

Back-end billing and collection work functions are those that are typically performed in a billing office. The work includes claims submission and claim edits, payment posting and cashiering, credit and refund processing, insurance follow-up, denial management, patient follow-up, and patient collections.

STAFFING DEPLOYMENT MODEL
FOR BILLING AND COLLECTION

The overall unit of work for a billing office is the insurance claim. The volume of claims determines the overall staff required to perform back-end billing functions. We expect approximately 10.00 staff full-time equivalents (FTE) per each 100,000 claims.[2] Most billing offices are organized by work function. A more detailed staffing analysis looks at the specific work function the staff in the billing office have been tasked to perform. The unit of work varies depending on the specific work function that has been delegated to the staff. For example, the unit of work for account follow-up staff is the number of accounts to be followed, and the unit of work for payment posting staff is the number of transactions and adjustments that are to be posted.

To build the staffing model for your billing office, follow the same steps we presented in earlier chapters of this book:

1. *Benchmark staff FTE and costs*

    Benchmarks are reported for "patient accounting" staff at the functional level in the MGMA *Cost Survey* instruments which is a portion of the overall staff category of "total business operations staff." Follow the staff benchmark process described in Chapter 4 to benchmark FTEs and cost for billing office staff.

2. *Evaluate staff workload*

    The unit of work for the staff is based on the specific job function the billing staff member has been tasked to perform. Workload ranges are available for each of the key billing functions of the revenue cycle and are reported in Exhibit 10.1. Use Chapter 5 as a guide to evaluate current staff workload and compare it to expected staff workload ranges for each key billing function.

---

[2] Walker Keegan, Deborah; Elizabeth W. Woodcock; and Sara M. Larch. 2009. *The Physician's Billing Process: 12 Potholes to Aviod in the Road to Getting Paid.* Englewood, Colo.: Medical Group Management Association.

3. *Redesign work processes*

   Redesign current work processes to streamline the work by minimizing waste and process handoffs and by standardizing work processes. Consider linking complementary work processes to minimize handoffs of the work from one staff member to the next and to provide staff with a work scope that is consistent with their knowledge and skills.

4. *Innovate your model*

   We describe a number of innovative models for staffing the revenue cycle. More ideas are provided in *The Physician Billing Process: 12 Potholes to Avoid in the Road to Getting Paid,* by Deborah Walker Keegan, Elizabeth W. Woodcock, Sara M. Larch (Medical Group Management Association, 2009).

PERFORMANCE EXPECTATIONS FOR BILLING AND COLLECTION

The performance workload ranges for each key billing function are listed in Chapter 5, The Staff Workload Evaluation Process, and are restated in Exhibit 10.1. Use these workload ranges to build the staffing model based on the actual work to be performed.

A number of factors influence the ability of staff to work within these ranges. These include the leverage of technology, the practice management system, the tools and processes required of the staff, the age and complexity of the accounts, and other similar factors. When issues of quantity versus quality arise, it is recommended that quality be the primary focus when identifying staff workload and performance.

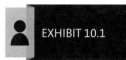

EXHIBIT 10.1	Expected Staff Workload Ranges for the Billing Office	

Work Function	Per Day	Per Hour
Charge entry line items without registration	375–525	55–75
Charge entry line items with registration	280–395	40–55
Payment and adjustment transactions posted manually	525–875	75–125
Insurance account follow-up, research and resolve by phone	N/A	6–12
Insurance account follow-up, research and resolve by appeal	N/A	3–4
Insurance account follow-up, check status of claim and rebill	N/A	12–60
Patient account follow-up	70–90	10–13

N/A = not applicable

Source: Walker Keegan, Deborah L.; Elizabeth W. Woodcock; and Sara M. Larch. 2009. *The Physician Billing Process: 12 Potholes to Avoid in the Road to Getting Paid.* Englewood, Colo.: Medical Group Management Association. Reprinted with permission.

The "Potholes" book contains additional expected staff workload ranges related to billing; the above figure reports a subset of these data.

INNOVATIVE STAFFING STRATEGIES FOR THE BILLING OFFICE

There are a number of staffing innovations to consider as you staff your billing office for optimal performance. These are described in the following paragraphs.

Develop Payer-Specific Knowledge

For front-end billing, staff based at the practice site need payer-specific knowledge so they can manage patient financial clearance, conduct accurate registration, obtain waiver forms, and collect time-of-service payments. For back-end billing, payer knowledge is critical for appropriate payment posting, account follow-up, and denial management. Each payer has its own rules and requirements related to coding and bundling, payment policies, denial and payment codes, and other important factors.

> For front-end billing, staff based at the practice site need payer-specific knowledge so they can manage patient financial clearance, conduct accurate registration, obtain waiver forms, and collect time-of-service payments.

Organize Insurance Account Follow-Up by Payer

We recommend that the insurance account follow-up staff be organized by payer. A payer may reject claims for coding or other reasons that may not be recognized early on if all staff are involved with all payers. This permits early identification of problem claims and problem payer performance. For large medical practices, an additional organizational level can be instituted along specialty categories, such as primary care, medical specialties, and surgical specialties. Within these levels, depending on the claim volume and claim complexity, a further delineation of staff can be made by service line. For example, within the insurance account follow-up unit there may be account follow-up staff devoted to a payer (such as Medicare) and then devoted to a specific specialty category (such as medical specialties) and then to a specific service line (such as cardiology). In this fashion, the medical practice delegates work on a functional basis with appropriate responsibility and defined accountability, combined with payer and specialty-specific knowledge.

Emphasize Front-End Billing

Historically, professional fee billing was considered a back-end process. Staff at the practice sites, including schedulers, check-in staff, clinical staff, and check-out staff, were not highly involved in the revenue cycle. Today, the key to a superior revenue cycle largely rests with these staff. They play a key role in obtaining complete registration and ensuring that payer-specific requirements are met, such as verifying and obtaining authorizations and waiver forms and meeting other required payer rules.

Though many medical practices have begun to recognize the enhanced and vital role played by staff outside of the traditional billing office, we believe that these staff will play an even greater role in the revenue cycle of the future. This is due to consumer-directed health plans and the need to collect higher levels of payments from patients in terms of deductibles, co-insurance, and copayments at time of service (if permitted by your contracts); the trend to collect patient responsibility payments prior to elective procedures and services; and the advent of real-time claims adjudication, where the information required by the payer to adjudicate the claim is entered at the point of care.

Thus, we believe that staffing the revenue cycle of the future (for non–hospital-based physicians) will largely rest with staff at the practice sites and with staff located in proximity to where the patient receives care. Indeed, many better-performing medical practices cite evidence that their investment in front-end billing has paid off, with higher percentages of clean claims being submitted and paid by payers. Doing it right the first time results in significantly fewer staffing resources being deployed for back-end billing functions and rework.

> Staffing the revenue cycle of the future will largely rest with staff at the practice sites and with staff located in proximity to where the patient receives care.

Link Complementary Work Functions

Consider linking functional work areas. Work linkages permit one staff member to have a broader breadth and scope of responsibility, and it minimizes work handoffs, improving staffing efficiency. Particularly with the increased volume of electronic payment remittance, linking payment posting and insurance account follow-up is a natural. Both tasks require in-depth, payer-specific knowledge in order to recognize under-profile payments and payer denial codes. Each task requires the staff to recognize and interpret the information the payer is attempting to convey through its explanation of benefits and various codes. Since both the payment posters and account follow-up staff require this same knowledge, many medical practices have adopted what is called total account ownership (TAO), which focuses the work of payment posting and insurance account follow-up with one individual responsible for a specific payer who is well versed in its nuances.[3] Care must be taken from an internal controls perspective to mitigate problems that might arise from one individual managing the entire account. However, with appropriate supervision, challenges to internal controls may be overcome.

Emphasize Process Dependency

All too often we have visited medical practices and have found that important work is simply waiting for a staff member to return from vacation or sick leave. The problem with this approach in staffing a revenue cycle is that process steps are highly interconnected and revenue can fluctuate at dangerous levels if one of the processes is significantly delayed. Therefore, we advocate a revenue cycle that is process-dependent rather than people-dependent. Staff need to be cross-trained in the medical practice to ensure that no key process simply waits.

When work is delayed in any key step in the revenue cycle, it has a profound impact on revenue and the medical practice's ability to

---

[3] Woodcock, Elizabeth W. 2007. "Total account ownership: A new model for streamlining your business office staff." *MGMA Connexion*. 7(1):28–33.

interpret and take action based on revenue cycle performance indi-
cators. As an example, let's suppose that the staff member assigned
to charge entry is on vacation for two weeks. Since charge entry is
needed for claims to be submitted, every back-end billing process
will be affected by this staff member's absence. Importantly, once
charge entry is brought to a current state, each staff member's workload, along the revenue cycle continuum, will exhibit high fluctuations. If management reports are produced during this same period,
the medical practice could mistakenly be alarmed at what it believes
is a significant decline in patient volume, when the problem is
simply due to the fact that no provisions were made to manage the
charge entry work in the employee's absence.

A process-dependent revenue cycle that involves staff who are cross-
trained not only helps you provide knowledge transfer throughout
the revenue cycle, but also reduces work fluctuations of staff and
revenue fluctuations for your medical practice.

Expand Work Scope

Cross-train staff for the work and expand the scope of their work.
For example, a staff member who manages account follow-up can
also work denials. A staff member who conducts registration functions can also work front-end claim edits. This permits staff to have a
full scope of work function and to be held fully accountable for that
work scope.

Build Checking into the Work

Billing audits are important in any medical practice. Beyond coding
and compliance audits, audits of the staff as they perform payment
posting, account adjustment, credit management, and account follow-up are needed to be sure the staff have the requisite knowledge
for the job.

In addition to these formal audits, build checking into the work
function. For example, if Andrea is assigned to work self-pay

accounts that have last names beginning with A through M, and Nancy is working N through Z, switch this work delegation at periodic intervals, for example, every three months. This built-in checking ensures that another set of eyes and talents are deployed to the work.

Prepare for New Payment Models

It is time now to prepare for new payment models. "Fee-for-service plus" reimbursement models are increasingly prevalent. For example, in addition to fee-for-service reimbursement, a medical practice may also receive pay-for-performance funding or care management fees. These types of reimbursement are likely to expand in the future, and staff need to be deployed to manage this reimbursement scheme.

KEY QUESTIONS TO ADDRESS AS YOU STAFF THE BILLING OFFICE

> ➤ Why are the staff performing at levels that vary from the expected range? There may be valid reasons a billing office appears to be overstaffed. If, for example, one of your primary payers is workers' compensation, which requires medical documentation at periodic intervals and other in-depth manual intervention, your billing office may require more staffing resources for billing and collection processes.

> ➤ Is the billing office leveraging technology to its fullest extent or are staff performing manual tasks that could be automated?

> ➤ Is there opportunity to improve the performance of the billing office? Do we have the right staff doing the right things consistent with the work?

> ➤ How many functions have been delegated to the staff? Is this multitasking impacting the efficiency of staff in performing any single function?

> ➤ Are the work processes to which the staff adhere encumbered or streamlined?

➤ Should we explore how other medical practices perform this function so we can learn new ways to improve the process?

➤ Does our billing system offer us the functionality that we need to perform at optimal levels? Are we using it appropriately? Do we deploy other technology available in the industry to leverage our human resources?

SUMMARY

In this chapter, we presented the key work functions for staff involved in billing and collection functions and the expected workload ranges of the staff based on work volume. Innovative staffing models for billing and collection activity include a decided emphasis on front-end billing and a payer-specific focus. As we discussed, your staff need to be actively engaged in the revenue cycle of your practice. You need the right staff doing the right things in order to achieve optimal revenue performance.

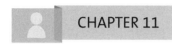

CHAPTER 11

Staffing for Medical Records and Electronic Health Records

Electronic health records are not simply electronic versions of the manual chart. To be effective, they need to be implemented as part of a patient flow redesign process involving changes to staffing models and patient access channels.

—Deborah Walker Keegan, PhD, FACMPE

One of the biggest mistakes in implementing electronic health records (EHRs) is a failure to redefine staff roles and work processes and to have the physician now do all the work!

In this chapter, we:

 ➤ Discuss changes to staff roles in medical practices with EHRs and due to meaningful use criteria for EHR incentive programs

 ➤ Measure and analyze the work of medical records staff

 ➤ Provide performance expectations for medical records staff

 ➤ Build a successful staffing model for medical records

 ➤ Share innovative staffing strategies for medical records support

 ➤ Provide key questions to address as you staff for medical records

CHANGES TO STAFF ROLES WITH EHRs

With the introduction of an EHR, the roles and responsibilities of support staff must change to ensure expanded patient access and physician productivity — and to ensure compliance with meaningful use criteria of the incentive programs for the adoption of EHRs.

Expanded Patient Access

EHRs open new patient access options for care. Patients can continue with face-to-face office visits, which are the traditional way care is provided, but they can also access the medical practice through a Web portal, virtual visits, secure messages, and home-directed care. When these access methods are available to patients, the staffing model in the medical practice must change to ensure that each patient access method is appropriately supported.

> With EHRs, a redesign of the patient flow process is needed to expand patient access and communication options. This requires a dramatic change to the current staffing deployment model of a medical practice.

Meaningful Use of EHRs

Given the meaningful use requirements of the government's EHR bonus payment program (as outlined in the American Recovery and Reinvestment Act of 2009, Title XIII Health Information Technology for Economic and Clinical Health Act, or HITECH Act), the roles of clinical support staff, in particular, need to be standardized and often expanded. To demonstrate meaningful use of EHRs, clinical staff need to assist physicians in using decision-support tools, tracking clinical conditions, collecting standardized data, and reporting clinical quality measures.

Stage one of the meaningful use requirements outlines 15 core measures and requires the selection of five measures from an additional menu that must be met in order to earn incentive payments for EHR implementation. Many of the core criteria require a change to the current patient flow process of a medical practice. For example, one core measure is to provide clinical summaries for patients for each office visit. This requires a change in clinical staff roles and responsibilities as well as monitoring to ensure compliance. Another core measure is to record and chart changes in specified vital signs in a structured fashion. This, too, requires that clinical staff be engaged in standardized work conducted in a systematic and formalized fashion.

Exhibit 11.1 summarizes the core measures required by the HI-TECH Act to demonstrate meaningful use of EHRs. As noted by this list, the clinical support staff are instrumental in assisting the physician to ensure that the criteria are met.

In addition, other members of the care team, such as the front office staff, can play a role in patient advocacy and patient activation, including reminding patients of upcoming clinical services consistent with disease and care registries and clinical protocols. It takes a dedicated team to provide the supportive infrastructure for clinical data and information capture, recording, and reporting.

As demonstrated by this discussion, a number of staffing changes should occur when an EHR is introduced. Re-evaluation of staff roles, skill needs, work processes, and transparency of work are needed, which results in a different staffing model for the medical practice.

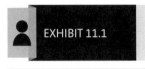

EXHIBIT 11.1	Meaningful Use Criteria Core Measurement Set*

1. Utilize computerized physician order entry

2. Implement drug-to-drug and drug-to-allergy interaction checks

3. Generate and transmit permissible prescriptions electronically (eR_X)

4. Record standard demographics as structured data

5. Maintain up-to-date problem list of current and active diagnoses

6. Maintain active medication list

7. Maintain active medication allergy list

8. Record and maintain vital signs as structured data

9. Record smoking status

10. Track and comply with one clinical decision-support rule relevant to specialty or high clinical priority

11. Report ambulatory clinical quality measures

12. Provide electronic copy of health information to patients upon request

13. Provide clinical summaries for patients for each office visit

14. Electronically exchange key clinical information among care providers and patient-authorized entities

15. Exercise technical capabilities to protect electronic health information

*The 15 core measures in this figure are significantly abbreviated. The full extent of the core measures and menu measures are available at http://edocket.access.gpo. gov/2010/pdf/2010-17207.pdf.

Changes to Work Processes

Due to the EHR, a number of different work processes need to be staffed. In medical practices without EHRs, patients telephone the practice to ask questions regarding their care and conditions, schedule visits, request lab and test results, request prescription renewals, and raise questions about their bills. In medical practices with EHRs, a Web portal permits patients to send electronic messages to the practice, with staff managing these messages throughout the day. Thus, staffing roles change to manage these online inquiries related to the clinical and business practice of medicine in lieu of telephone calls. These changing work processes are summarized in Exhibit 11.2.

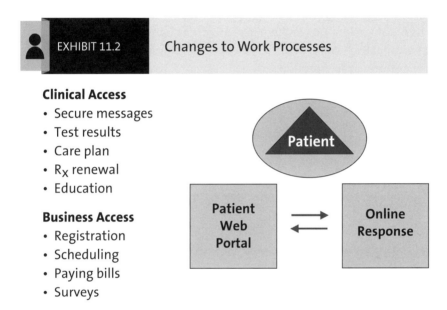

EXHIBIT 11.2   Changes to Work Processes

Clinical Access
- Secure messages
- Test results
- Care plan
- R_X renewal
- Education

Business Access
- Registration
- Scheduling
- Paying bills
- Surveys

Patient

Patient Web Portal

Online Response

These new work processes must be staffed once a Web portal is introduced. A Web portal must be supported to permit electronic interchange with patients. This is a new work process for many medical practices; it needs to be staffed so the practice can interact with patients across multiple access channels for clinical care and business-of-medicine functions.

Changes to Clinical Support

With EHRs, the skill mix of staff needs to change to reflect differences in infrastructure and support to the physician. In particular, telephone nursing is facilitated due to the proximity and direct access to the patient's medical record. No longer is a message taken, the medical record pulled, the message and chart transported to the nurse, with the nurse phoning the patient to obtain additional information and finally, responding to the patient's needs. With EHRs, inbound calls of a clinical nature can be handled by clinical staff with immediate access to the record. This streamlines the work associated with the external patient flow process and also permits the patient to receive information in an expedited fashion. This change to managing clinical calls permits medical practices to respond to patients within 30 minutes, a turnaround time suggested by many as appropriate.

When EHRs are fully leveraged, nursing staff have access to the chart and can be deployed in different roles. Staff roles to manage telephone triage, nurse advice, virtual visits, and community and remote access through telemedicine, outreach care, case management, and health and wellness coaching are all facilitated by the availability of online medical records. These changes are shown in Exhibit 11.3.

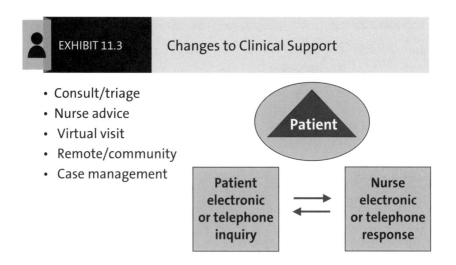

EXHIBIT 11.3   Changes to Clinical Support

- Consult/triage
- Nurse advice
- Virtual visit
- Remote/community
- Case management

Patient

Patient electronic or telephone inquiry → ← Nurse electronic or telephone response

Changes to the Patient Visit

Support for the patient visit and the patient visit itself changes with the adoption of EHRs.

Patient Visit Support

One of the errors some medical practices make when they implement EHRs is to discontinue requiring the nurse or medical assistant to prepare in advance for the visit. After all, they say, the physician now has access to the chart and can conduct this piece of work independently. Medical practices that take this position have effectively delegated work upward from the nurse to the physician, which is the entirely incorrect direction we want to take if we are striving for physician and practice efficiency.

Instead, those who correctly implement EHRs actually build in more steps for the clinical support staff. These additional steps include anticipating physician needs and care interventions for patients. The work includes providing enhanced direct patient care during the visit by preparing the patient for the provider, providing patient education, and discharging the patient from the exam room. With EHRs, a summary of the visit and a summary of the care and treatment plan can be provided to the patient at discharge from the exam room. This document serves as a take-home reference and aids the patient in self-management. Note that a clinical summary provided to patients is also one of the core measures in the meaningful use criteria for EHR adoption. The clinical support staff of the medical practice play an active role in providing this document to the patient and in reviewing the critical aspects of the patient's current and subsequent care and treatment plan.

Virtual Visits

With EHRs, medical practices have worked to expand their online consults and virtual visits: visits that occur in a non–face-to-face fashion. This includes telephone visits, e-consults, e-visits, and secure online message threads between the care team and the patient. The clinical support staff plays an added role in this virtual environment by supporting the physician in the management of this electronic exchange.

Managing the Inbox

When EHRs are introduced in a medical practice, the physician's inbox is like a living, breathing appendage. It expands and contracts daily; at first glance, physicians often feel overwhelmed, given its size. Again, a change to staff work functions permits physicians to manage this new work input. When preparing for the patient visit, the nurse should review the electronic chart and prepare for the visit. The physician can review the schedule prior to the visit and send an e-instruction to the nurse. The nurse can separate normal from abnormal test results, similar to a manual categorization of test results into two piles, with flagging of abnormal tests for the physician's initial focus.

Managing the inbox is really an issue of staging. Should the physician do it all, should the nurse first work the inbox and flag items for the physician, or should there be a shared inbox involving the physician and nurse, with the physician huddling with the nurse at established intervals during the day to jointly work the box? This decision and its impact on current staffing and skill mix requirements needs to be addressed as part of implementing EHRs in the medical practice and determining the appropriate staffing strategy consistent with the EHR implementation.

> When EHRs are introduced in a medical practice, the physician's inbox is like a living, breathing appendage. Staff need to be deployed to assist with this work.

Clinical Preparation for the Visit

Preparation for the patient visit also needs to occur differently when EHRs are used. For new patients, their history, background, and referral records need to be entered into the electronic record. In some medical practices, this is done by medical records staff, in others it is done by schedulers, in others it revolves around the clinical support staff, and in still others it is delegated to the patient (with an electronic upload of his or her data to the medical record). Regardless of who is delegated this responsibility, the goal should be to populate the EHR in advance of the patient visit so the physician has the information needed to make the initial visit with the patient meaningful.

Medication Documentation

The clinical support staff should be given an expanded role in medication documentation. At each visit, the medication list should be updated from a drop-down menu of options, with reasons provided for discontinuation of medications as appropriate. Physicians often indicate that the work involved in creating an up-to-date list of medications is one of the toughest challenges with an EHR, due to the considerable time and effort required. The physician can be supported in this process by educated clinical staff with well-defined boundaries regarding the capture and recording of current and discontinued medications for the patient.

Concurrent Visit Steps

It is important to recognize that with EHRs, the patient visit does not need to continue to consist of a set of sequential steps. Instead, concurrent steps to the visit can be taken. For example, the physician and the nurse can enter the exam room together, with the nurse documenting the exam based on the physician's oral reports, assisting with the visit, and providing end of visit education and discharge instructions. We have observed multiple instances where the physician enters the exam room and repeats the questions that the nurse has already posed to the patient. This is an example of a sequential process gone awry.

It is important to recognize that with EHRs, the patient visit does not need to continue to consist of a set of sequential steps.

Additional changes in the role of clinical support staff due to EHRs are summarized in Exhibit 11.4. As this demonstrates, there are real changes involving physician instruction, patient inquiries, patient-specific protocols, and test and laboratory results reporting.

 EXHIBIT 11.4   Changing Role of Clinical Support Staff

Separate internal and external patient visit support	Telephone nurse/Web portal support; nurse patient-visit support
Physician instruction to nurse	Instant messaging/inbox message to nurse
Physician/nurse instruction to patient	Electronic message to patient
Patient inquiries	Inquiries maintained in running lists, proactive management with patient, use of charts and graphs to assist patient self-management and activation
Patient-specific protocols	Managed by nurse and physician; patient self-management and reporting
Procedure and test results	Electronic patient recall, online results via Web portal
Documentation	Scribes; expanded nurse charting roles involving structured data

Scribes

A number of medical practices recognize that EHRs permit consolidated storage of patient information and enhanced access to data and information for care and treatment, yet they often are also found to slow down the busy physician — particularly when the EHR is initially introduced. In these situations and in specialties that require the physician to use equipment as part of the patient visit, scribes are often introduced to document key aspects of the patient visit. For example, a busy dermatologist who is conducting a full-body exam on a patient will often have a scribe in the room to record the size of moles and other discolorated or raised areas. As another example, the busy ophthalmologist who examines patients using various types of eye equipment will often have a scribe to record the findings of the examination. More and more medical practices use scribes — often a medical assistant or nurse — to improve physician efficiency. Many physicians in orthopedic surgery, family medicine, and pediatrics use scribes in their medical practices, evidence that this approach is expanding beyond the traditional specialties that have employed them in the past.

In academic medical practices, nonphysician providers often serve as scribes. In these settings, the nonphysician provider may dictate or document the physician's note as part of the physician/nonphysician provider covisit with the patient. This saves considerable time for a busy faculty member and often leads to more detailed patient documentation than can be attempted by a faculty member who is typically providing clinical care part-time, given his or her other teaching and research activities.

Patient Outreach

EHRs have also permitted medical practices to transition from a "build it and they will come" mentality to a patient outreach mentality. In these practices, clinical staff are assigned to work via electronic registries and recall systems to reach out to patients in a care or case management role. This helps the patient comply with his or her care and treatment plan. It also reduces inbound telephone calls, inappropriate admissions, and inappropriate visits. Instead, a nurse reaches out to patients to determine their status and responds to their questions and concerns. More formal programs involving this type of outreach use health and wellness coaches to work with groups of patients based on diagnosis or type of intervention, such as recent hospital discharge. A further discussion of the changing roles for nursing staff is presented in Chapter 12, Staffing the Medical Home Model.

Patient Activation

More and more frequently, medical practices are working to activate patients to maintain or improve their health and wellness. There are a number of technologies that can be used to help patients become more engaged. These include Web portals, patient health records, patient logs and journals, an electronic medication summary, an after-visit summary, online tools, videos, and graphs. Through these tools, patients are encouraged to become active, rather than passive, participants in their own care and are encouraged to be more accountable for their own behavior and actions. Staff involvement in each technology needs to be defined in a medical practice. The currency of the technology, the monitoring and oversight of the information shared with patients, the response to the patients' inquiries and contributions to their records, and other similar work must be formally assigned to staff in the medical practice.

WORK FUNCTIONS OF MEDICAL RECORDS STAFF

Medical practices that continue to use manual medical charts staff their medical records unit differently than those with EHRs. Key work functions for each type of medical records unit include:

> ➤ *Manual medical records.* Sorting patient materials by name or number; pulling charts; filing; refiling; locating charts; responding to inbound faxes, e-mails, telephone and online requests for chart pulls; linking charts to inbound requests

(for example, telephone messages and fax prescription renewals from pharmacy); medical records-release functions (for example, to patient, another provider, insurance company, attorney)

➤ *EHRs.* Scanning outside records to the medical practice's EHR, including links to appropriate tabs and placement in the EHR; data input of clinical records; oversight of electronic inboxes to ensure timeliness and completeness; medical records-release functions

In some medical practices, the medical records staff are also involved in:

➤ Completing a portion of forms based on information in the medical records, such as disability forms

➤ Carrying out physician requests regarding medical records information, such as sending letters regarding normal laboratory results to patients

➤ Monitoring logs to ensure that dictated transcription is received, signed, and sent to the appropriate parties

➤ Transcribing physician visit notes and letters to referring physicians (this role has been phased out in many of today's medical practice, particularly those with EHRs)

PERFORMANCE EXPECTATIONS FOR MEDICAL RECORDS STAFF

Not only are the work functions different, but also the performance expectations for the quantity of work to be performed are different in a medical practice with electronic records as compared to those with manual charts. In both types of medical practices, however, quality is vitally important to ensure that records are filed in the correct charts and in the correct location in the charts to facilitate quality patient care.

Manual Medical Records

Highly productive medical practices with manual medical records typically employ .35 full-time equivalent (FTE) medical records staff per FTE physician. Based on function, we typically expect 1.00 staff FTE to be able to pull and/or refile 140 to 175 charts per day. Another measure used to determine the staffing needs for a medical practice with manual charts is annual patient visit volume. Staffing the medical records unit based on patient visit volume is typically built as 1.00 staff FTE required for every 13,000 to 15,000 patient visits. If your medical practice has 30,000 annual patient visits, we would thus expect a range of 2.00 FTE to 2.30 FTE medical records staff.

Electronic Health Records

To determine the number of medical records staff required to scan records into the EHR, determine the approximate time it takes to conduct this work, then assume a seven-hour productive day and identify an expected workload range consistent with this analysis. For example, if it takes your staff five minutes to scan new patient paperwork, then it is reasonable to expect a staff workload from 75 to 95 new patient packets scanned per day (calculated as 7 hours × 60 minutes per hour = 420 minutes; 420 minutes divided by 5 minutes equals 84; range set at approximately 10 units lower and 10 higher than the range).

BUILDING A STAFF MODEL FOR MEDICAL RECORDS

To build a successful staffing model for medical records functions, follow the same steps presented in earlier chapters.

1. *Benchmark staff FTEs and costs*

   Follow the steps in Chapter 4 to benchmark the number and cost of your medical records staff to MGMA *Cost Survey* instruments. The functional staff level of "medical records" is reported in the survey instrument, which is a subset of the categorical staffing level of "total front office support staff."

2. *Evaluate staff workload*

   Follow the steps in Chapter 5 to perform a gap analysis between current work quantity performed and expected staff workload ranges associated with medical records functions. Identify the number of loose papers and the number of files that need to be pulled and refiled (for manual records) and the number of documents to be scanned (for electronic records) for a representative week in order to conduct this analysis.

3. *Redesign work processes*

   Determine the scope of work to be performed by the medical records staff. For example, are they sorting records to be filed or are they actually filing the records? What is the extent of work associated with looking for the chart? How many work handoffs are involved in message-taking, faxes, and subsequent chart pulls? Then redesign the work to streamline the process and reduce waste and non–value-added process steps.

4. *Innovate your model*

INNOVATIVE STRATEGIES FOR MEDICAL PRACTICES WITH MANUAL MEDICAL RECORDS

Explore the following innovations for staffing a manual medical records unit.

Standardize Courier Functions

Use online chart request methods. Staff can pull the charts and deliver them to the practice site at established times throughout the day, for example, 10:00 a.m., 12:00 p.m., 2:00 p.m., and 4:00 p.m., unless charts are urgently needed.

Reduce Process Steps

Print the pharmacy faxes and telephone messages in the medical records unit, with staff pulling the charts and delivering both chart and message simultaneously, thereby reducing work handoffs and time required by the nurse to link the chart with the message.

Track Medical Records

Use a formal system to track the chart — for example, a bar code or outguide transfer process.

Establish Expectations for Timely Filing

Expect records to be filed within 24 hours of receipt.

Create Formal Work Assignments

Rather than expect all staff to do every work process each day, segment the work into discrete work units and formally assign a specific unit of work to the staff to perform. Some examples include:

- Separately assign sorting of loose papers, filing, pulling of charts, refiling, and courier functions to increase staff efficiency.

- Consider rotating staff roles to provide work variation and cross-training.

- Assign staff by medical record number (or patient last name alpha) when they are filing/refiling. This assists in identifying errors specific to a staff member, thereby ensuring accountability for work performance.

- Create a closed-loop process for transcription receipt and filing. This involves the use of a spreadsheet or other recording method to ensure that all material sent for transcription was received by the office and has been approved by the physician prior to filing. Medical records staff can also be involved in mailing normal laboratory results to patients once they are reviewed and approved by the physician.

➤ Ensure complete and accurate logs for medical release. A designated staff member in the medical practice should manage this function centrally, given the specific regulations related to medical release, with logs and records maintained for each release.

KEY QUESTIONS TO ADDRESS AS YOU STAFF FOR MEDICAL RECORDS

Electronic Health Records

➤ What changes in staffing roles are required now that the medical practice has electronic records?

➤ What changes to the patient flow process should be made to expand patient access and communication methods?

➤ With EHRs, can work be co-located and/or performed remotely by a central staff unit?

➤ What additional work should be delegated to clinical support staff and to front office staff?

Manual Charts

➤ What is the scope of work delegated to the staff? Is this delegation efficient or is there a better way to manage the work?

➤ Can processes be streamlined? For example, with manual charts, is there a less labor-intensive way to locate charts throughout the practice? As another example, can fax requests and telephone messages be printed in the medical records area, with charts pulled and attached to the message prior to being sent to the back-office nurse for management?

➤ Can the work be focused based on time? For example, can charts for telephone messages be pulled throughout the day and couriered to the practice suites at established times throughout the day (unless it is an urgent issue)?

➤ Can the work be divided into segments to improve efficiency? For example, can some staff be assigned to sort loose papers for filing, with others filing and refiling charts, and others performing courier functions?

➤ What additional roles can the medical records staff play as part of the care team?

SUMMARY

In this chapter, we discussed the importance of redesigning the patient flow process and staffing models of a medical practice when EHRs are introduced. The specific work functions and tasks for staff change to effectively leverage the EHR with patient flow. The role of medical records staff continues to change and the traditional roles have expanded, with these staff serving a more prominent role on the care team.

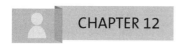

CHAPTER 12

Staffing the Medical Home Model

Because the Medical Home is gaining traction, AND if the government reform initiative incorporates the medical home AND if the payer community begins to pay a differential to an accredited medical home, there will be a stampede for most primary care physician settings to become accredited as Medical Homes.

—Marshall M. Baker, MS, FACMPE, President/CEO
Physician Advisory Services, Inc.

The patient-centered medical home is receiving attention as a promising new primary care delivery model to improve quality and reduce cost. Medical home demonstration projects are in process, and the future of medical homes depends upon their ability to successfully demonstrate value (defined as high quality and low cost) amid the overall landscape of healthcare reform.

The staffing strategy for a medical home is very different from that of a traditional medical practice. It typically involves higher levels of nursing staff, in particular. In this chapter, we:

- Define the medical home model
- Discuss staffing roles for the care team
- Determine workload expectations for the care team

DEFINITION OF THE PATIENT-CENTERED MEDICAL HOME MODEL

In a medical home model, patients are assigned to a personal care physician and the physician and care team provide access and outreach to patients on a 24/7 basis. The intent of this model is to provide assistance to the patient to maintain health and wellness and, at the same time, minimize costly care, such as that provided in an urgent care or emergency room facility. Care is coordinated not only with specialists and over the transitions of care (primary to specialty to hospital to home to nursing home), but also with caregivers, to include family members and others who provide support to the patient.

> In a medical home model, patients are assigned to a personal care physician, and the physician and care team provide access and outreach to patients on a 24/7 basis.

A medical home is a medical practice that caters to the patient in a unique way. The key components of the medical home include the following:

→ *Personal physician:* A personal physician is assigned to each patient and is the team leader for a support staff who are collectively responsive to the patient and patient's family or caregiver for comprehensive care.

→ *Access to care:* Multiple access channels are available to the patient to meet his or her healthcare needs. These include expanded access for face-to-face visits with the personal physician and team members, 24/7 access to the care team, and virtual visits involving telephone, e-mail, and other mobile health and telehealth exchanges with patients and caregivers.

→ *Transitions of care:* The team coordinates transitions of care and provides for all of the patient's health needs. Transitions of care from primary to specialty to hospital to home to nursing home are managed in a well-coordinated and seamless manner. The coordination of care is facilitated by clinical information systems, registries, telehealth, and other modalities to ensure timely and appropriate care for the patient.

> ➤ *Quality focus:* Quality and safety are paramount in a medical home model, with evidence-based and clinical decision-making tools used in a systematic approach to provide the right care to the patient. Patients are actively involved in shared decision-making regarding their care and treatment plan and are active in self-management, with tools and resources provided to patients to permit their activation and engagement.

Coordination of care is facilitated by clinical information systems, registries, telehealth, and other modalities to ensure timely and appropriate care for the patient.

Recognizing that this approach to care requires a financial model different from traditional fee-for-service reimbursement, medical homes are typically paid on a "fee-for-service plus" basis; traditional reimbursement is supplemented by a care or case management fee. Patient-centered medical homes have demonstrated improvement to patient health indices and reduced costs associated with reductions in emergency room visits, admissions for ambulatory-sensitive conditions, and other similar costly interventions. Quality and cost measures maintained by medical home models often extend beyond the level of a unique patient to that of a patient population.

STAFFING STRATEGIES FOR THE MEDICAL HOME MODEL

If patient-centered medical homes become the preferred primary care delivery system for the future, it is important to understand the staffing models and strategies needed to ensure success. The organizations that have demonstrated proven success with these models have a heightened involvement of clinical support staff, including registered nurses (RNs), licensed practical nurses (LPNs), and medical assistants (MAs). In addition, patients in medical homes appear to be more actively engaged in their care. They become extensions of the medical practice staff by using online systems to schedule appointments, request prescription renewals, obtain laboratory and test results, update information, and initiate inquiries to the medical practice.

> The organizations that have demonstrated success with medical home models have a heightened involvement of clinical support staff. In addition, patients in medical homes appear to be more actively engaged in their care.

Although each patient-centered medical home model embraces common elements, there is no single delivery model that has been adopted for today's medical home. For example:

➤ *Medical Home Model A:* Emphasizes face-to-face visits with the physician, supplementing these with nurse case management outreach to a select subset of patients via telephone.

➤ *Medical Home Model B:* Works to reduce the volume of face-to-face visits with the patient; however, extends the time of these visits to ensure a comprehensive examination. Supplements the in-person visit with virtual visits, including telephone encounters and secure online messaging with the care team.

As we have demonstrated in this book, staffing models are developed around the quantity and type of work to be performed. Thus, there is no single staffing deployment model for today's medical home. The following caregivers are typically found in a medical home or the patient is directly connected to one of these caregivers as appropriate.

Physician

The physician in a medical home does not necessarily need to be a primary care physician. However, the physician needs to assume a "whole-person" orientation toward the patient. For example, an obstetrician gynecologist, infectious disease physician, or noninvasive cardiologist could likely qualify if he or she assumes all of the internal medicine services of the patient.

The panel size, which is conservatively defined as the unique patients seen by a physician within a 12-month period, varies depending on the medical home model that is adopted. Consistent with our example earlier:

> *Medical Home Model A:* The physician may have a panel size of 2,300 to 2,500, schedule patients for 9 or 10 clinical sessions per week, providing face-to-face patient access 36 to 40 hours per week, and seeing 24 to 32 patients per day. This is supplemented by a planned approach toward after-hours and weekend care, as well as case management and outreach.

> *Medical Home Model B:* The physician may have a panel size of 1,800 to 2,000 and only have face-to-face visits with 12 to 15 patients per day, yet there is a shift in work from face-to-face visits to virtual visits by telephone and online, secure messages with the patient.[1] A formal, planned approach to provide care and resources to the patient 24/7 supplements this and extends patient access to care.

Staffing for Telephones, Front Office, and Visit Support

To determine the staffing model for the face-to-face visits in the medical home model and for the telephone support needed to meet

---

[1] Group Health of Puget Sound has published the outcomes of its medical home model, which combines face-to-face visits with virtual visits involving a reduction in physician panel size. See: Reid, Robert J.; Katie Coleman; Eric A. Johnson; et al. 2010. "The group health medical home at year two: Cost savings, higher patient satisfaction, and less burnout for physicians." *Health Affairs.* 29(5):835–843.

patient inbound demand, employ the tools and approaches described in Chapter 7, Staffing the Telephones; Chapter 8, Staffing the
Front Office; and Chapter 9, Staffing the Visit.

Building the staff model based on the expected staff workload ranges
associated with each work function is an appropriate model that recognizes both the work function and the quantity of work performed
by members of the medical home care team.

Beyond these more typical support staff, a medical home model has
a care team focused on the well-being of the patient, the patient's
family, and caregivers.

THE CARE TEAM

The physician-led care team is comprised of a combination of the
following members. Note that these are not mutually exclusive, that
is, one or more of the functions may be combined (for example, a
care manager may also serve as a transition manager).

Nonphysician Providers

One or more advanced practice nurses or other nonphysician providers may leverage the physician as part of the care team. Their role
varies based on the work assigned. (See Chapter 15, Role Options for
Nonphysician Providers, for a discussion of these roles.)

Virtual Nurse

The care team typically includes a licensed nurse who manages
inbound telephone calls from patients and conducts triage and
advice. The nurse typically responds to secure online messages from
patients, first screening the messages and either responding to them
within the scope of licensure and delegation or sending them to the
physician or nonphysician provider for resolution and response.
This nurse also contacts patients with laboratory and test results, or
patients obtain these results online via a patient Web portal.

Care Manager

Care managers are typically licensed nurses who manage a panel of patients. Patients identified as high-risk based on their condition or disease state, have multiple chronic care conditions, or who need outreach support are assigned to a care manager. The care manager typically contacts the patient one or more times per month to discuss the patient's current status and provide education and resources specific to the patient's condition.

Nurse Navigator or Transition Manager

A nurse navigator or transition manager is typically a licensed nurse or other qualified staff who is focused on managing transitions of care. For example, a patient may need to see a specialist. This transition manager provides patient information to the specialist and coordinates records flow and scheduling. Similarly, this staff member is involved in hospital admission for the patient and transfer from hospital to home care, providing a seamless transition.

Health and Wellness Coach

The licensure and skill level of a health and wellness coach depends on the type of coaching performed. For example, a wellness coach may reach out to a patient who has adopted a weight loss program to ensure he or she is on track. A health coach may reach out to patients who are on certain medications, ensuring they are taking them as prescribed and reviewing any side effects they are having. With today's technology, health and wellness coaches are increasingly involved in electronic reminders to patients, such as sending text messages to patients to remind them of their blood pressure checks, glucose monitoring, and other self-care aids.

Clinical Pharmacist

A clinical pharmacist is assigned to patients to review medication management, side effects, and refill and renewal activity. The pharmacist may also be involved in anticoagulation management and other similar long-term medication management for the patient. The pharmacist is a valuable member of the care team, helping patients manage their medications and thereby improving physician efficiency specifically for patients taking multiple medications, suffering multiple chronic care conditions, or who have medication, allergies or other sensitivities.

Social Worker

A social worker may be called in to work with patients, families, and caregivers to ensure a smooth transition for patients to home care and/or to identify community resources to benefit patients.

Psychologist or Psychiatrist

Consistent with the whole-person orientation of medical home models, a psychologist or psychiatrist may be involved with patients to assist them in meeting episodic or chronic mental health challenges.

Alternative Medicine

Supplementing traditional, Western medicine is Chinese medicine, such as acupuncture, as well as other alternative therapies. These are consistent with the whole-person orientation specific to the patient and the patient's condition.

WORKLOAD EXPECTATIONS FOR THE CARE TEAM

Today's medical home models typically have 1.5 to 1.75 full-time equivalents (FTEs) clinical support staff per FTE physician.[2] However, the number and skill mix of staff vary based on how the medical home is defined and the services that are provided. If a medical home

---

[2] See Kuzel, Anton J. 2009. "Ten steps to a patient-centered medical home." *Family Practice Management.* www.aafp.org/online/en/home/publications/journals/fpm/ preprint/kuzel.printerviewhtml/. Accessed 1/23/10.

anticipates patient needs by providing information and outreach to the patient, a different staffing model will be required from one that focuses on bringing patients to the practice for face-to-face visits. In most medical homes, however, we see higher levels of nursing and/or medical assistant support to manage the various access channels for patients and to conduct the care management and outreach functions typical of these delivery systems.

Group Health of Puget Sound in Washington has published extensively on the composition and outcomes of its medical home model. Its staffing model is specific to the type of work functions employed by the care team, with approximately 30 percent of primary care visits currently provided via virtual medicine. Its staffing levels for clinical support staff in its medical home model are 1.20 FTE RNs, 2.00 FTE LPNs, and 5.60 FTE MAs for every 10,000 patients. Group Health also provides extensive access channels for patients via a patient Web portal, a consulting nurse service that is available 24/7, and other similar support.[3]

Following are examples of the type and quantity of work expected of specific care team members often found in the patient-centered medical home model of care.

Virtual Nurse

A virtual nurse takes and responds to inbound telephone calls from patients and also typically manages secure online messages sent by patients. The volume of work expected is 65 to 85 calls and inquiries per day, or eight to 12 per hour, which is five to eight minutes per inquiry (assuming a seven-hour productive day) (as reported in Exhibit 5.3). The nurse may reside in the medical practice or alternatively, work from a remote location with access to the electronic health record.

---

[3] Source: Reid, Robert J.; Katie Coleman; Eric A. Johnson; et al. 2010. "The group health medical home at year two: Cost savings, higher patient satisfaction, and less burnout for physicians." *Health Affairs.* 29(5):835–843.

Care Manager and Transition Manager

To guide the patient's care, a staff member may be tasked with a combination of the care and transition manager roles. A RN trained in guided care nursing works with three to five physicians to care for 50 to 60 complex, chronically ill patients. The RN is involved in developing a care guide and action plan for patients, reaches out to patients on a monthly or more frequent basis, assesses patients at home, and is involved in transitions of care, patient self-management, and identifying community resources for patients.[4]

Health and Wellness Coach Models

The workload for health coaches depends on the type of coaching they provide. Caseloads are highly variable based on type and approach. In a recent survey, 36 percent of the coaches were assigned 100 or more patients; however, there was generally an equal distribution among the other caseload ranges (one to 24 patients, 25 to 49 patients, and 50 to 99 patients at approximately 20 percent each).[5]

A health coach will typically be on the phone six to seven hours per day, four to five days per week, with many of the coaches working from home rather than residing in the medical practice.[6]

The following types of coaches are provided today by health plans and, increasingly, by medical practices. A care team member in the

---

[4] The phrase *guided care* was developed at Johns Hopkins University. See www.guidedcare.org for more information on this model. The work functions and expectations were presented by Dr. Chad Boult, Professor of Public Health, Medicine and Nursing at Johns Hopkins University at the National Medical Home Summit, Philadelphia, Pennsylvania, March 3, 2009.

[5] Health coach caseloads are reported in the *Healthcare Intelligence Network, 2010 Health Coaching Benchmarks: Operations and Performance Data for Optimal Program ROI and Participant Health Status.* Based on 2009 HIN Health & Wellness Coaching Survey. Report available at www.him.com and www.hin.com/chartoftheweek/health_coaching_monthly_caseload. Accessed 11/10/2010.

[6] Ibid.

medical home model is often assigned to provide this type of support to the patient[7]:

> *Laser coach:* Focuses on disease management and performs brief patient interventions typically 10 to 20 minutes long.

> *Wellness coach:* Focuses on the patient's physical and mental health needs.

> *Health coach:* Focuses on the health and medical needs of the patient.

> *Fitness coach:* Assists patients with lifestyle choices, including nutrition and physical fitness.

REIMAGINE THE PATIENT VISIT

In today's medical home models, the focus is not on increasing the quantity of face-to-face visits (which is often the focus for medical practices with traditional fee-for-service reimbursement). Picture a new model:

> The patient calls her care team to describe a health issue.

> The physician orders a laboratory test that same day.

> The patient goes to a local laboratory for testing during her lunch break from work.

> The results of the test are e-mailed or telephoned to the patient that same day and she is instructed to go for an ultrasound.

> The ultrasound scheduler e-mails the patient and/or calls her to schedule the ultrasound for the next day (or the patient logs in to a Website and schedules the procedure).

> The results of the ultrasound are communicated to the patient the same day via e-mail or telephone call.

---

[7] Ibid.

In a traditional medical practice, this episode of care with the patient would involve multiple face-to-face visits and significant delays. In a medical home model, prompt response is a daily occurrence, with efforts expended to reduce even this limited number of process steps.

SUMMARY

In this chapter, we described the patient-centered medical home model and the various roles care team members play when assuming a whole-person orientation to the patient. We contrasted this with a traditional medical practice that does not have the extended team members involved in the patient's course of care. Consistent with the approach we have taken in this book, the staff work function and work volume dictate the number and skill mix of staff needed for the medical home care team, with the staffing deployment model built consistent with the work.

PART 4

Innovative Strategies to Optimize Flexibility and Leverage Physicians

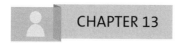

CHAPTER 13

Staffing Models for Fluctuating Work Levels and Other Realities

Stuff happens in a medical practice.

—Bruce A. Johnson, JD, MPA
Health Lawyer and Consultant

Despite best intentions, things don't always proceed as smoothly as we would hope in a medical practice. It is not possible to anticipate each and every situation and, at times, the staff need to think on their feet to respond to daily operational challenges. An area that we can plan for, however, is fluctuating work volumes. We can work to match the staffing levels with the work to be performed. We can also try to optimize the use of the practice space, recognizing that a reduction in per-unit visit costs will help the bottom line of the medical practice. And we can ensure that the important work of a medical practice is attended to, even if the practice has a shortage of staff for a defined period of time.

In this chapter, we describe:

- ➤ Staffing to meet fluctuating work volume
- ➤ Staffing to optimize facility utilization
- ➤ Work segmentation strategies
- ➤ Work extension strategies
- ➤ Work rotation strategies

STAFFING TO MEET FLUCTUATING WORK VOLUME

In many medical practices, physicians are not present in the office setting five days per week, two four-hour sessions per day. Patient visit volume fluctuates by day of week and session per day. The work of staff members involved in the patient visit is therefore variable, consistent with the visit volume fluctuations.

> With fluctuating patient visit volume, a static staffing model means that the medical practice will either overstaff or understaff for the work.

Many medical practices incur a high staffing cost because they are not actually staffing for the work. In these medical practices, staff are assigned a static schedule, such as 8:00 a.m. to 5:00 p.m., regardless of the volume of work to be performed. If the physician is in surgery, rounding at the hospital, or at meetings, the same number of staff is assigned to their roles day-in and day-out. Similarly, regardless of inbound telephone demand, medical practices will err in their staffing model by assigning the same number of people to manage the telephones, whether it is Monday morning when the phones ring off the hook, or Wednesday afternoon when the phones are silent.

The consequences of this static staffing pattern are that the staff are not able to meet patient demand or provide the infrastructure and support to the physician in a logical, planned approach. Instead, on certain days and during certain sessions of the day, there are more or fewer staff than are required to adequately provide the infrastructure and support for a streamlined patient flow process. Another consequence is the cost of overtime. When there is insufficient staffing for the work, a medical practice may incur significant overtime — and poor patient satisfaction. By planning for these work variations, a more appropriate — and less costly — staffing pattern can be deployed.

By adopting a variable staffing model instead of a static model, medical practices can link the appropriate number and type of staff for the work. A number of variable staffing strategies are available to medical practices. These are summarized in Exhibit 13.1 and further described in the following sections.

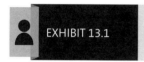 **EXHIBIT 13.1**   Staffing Strategies to Support Fluctuating Work Levels

Strategy	Description
Staff assignments by clinic session	Staff assigned by clinic session based on anticipated work volume
Consolidated work	Work consolidated with a few staff, with the others reassigned or scheduled home
Voluntary time off or send-off	Staff volunteer to go home or are scheduled off
Part-time or per-diem staff	Part-time staff scheduled for peak demand to supplement full-time staff
Medical practice assistants	Staff have an expanded work scope and skills in order to flexibly manage multiple clinical and business functions
Internal float pool	Staff are hired in anticipation of leave trends and staff vacancies. The pool of workers is fully trained to the medical practice's technology and work processes
Multitasking	Limited cross-training of staff for specific peak periods

(Continued on next page)

Strategy	Description
Nurse leverage	Nurse takes patient history and presents the patient to the physician, improving the quality of patient history and reducing physician face-to-face visit time, while providing team care to the patient*
Volunteers	Community volunteers augment the role of employed staff for basic functions, such as reception and scanning of medical records

*Anderson, Peter, and Marc D. Halley. 2008 "A new approach to making your doctor–nurse team more productive." *Fam Pract Manag.* 15(17):35–40.

Staff Assignments by Clinic Session

In medical practices that have adopted a staff-per-clinic-session strategy, a supervisor reviews the appointment schedules, trends inbound calls, and other indices and determines the staffing assignments required for individual clinic sessions based on the anticipated work. The staffing assignments thus change daily depending on the work variation.

Consolidated Work

In this strategy, work is consolidated with a select number of staff in order to ensure a full complement of work. For example, rather than having each nurse continue to work in the suite when their physician is out of the office in order to simply manage a low volume of inbound telephone calls from patients, the work is consolidated with one or two nurses who perform this work full-time, with the others scheduled to be off or assigned other roles and responsibilities. If this staff model works when the physician is out of the office it should also be considered for use as a permanent model. A telephone nurse triage unit manages inbound telephone calls rather than each physician's nurse in the practice.

Voluntary Time Off or Send-Off

In medical practices with a time-off or send-off strategy, the supervisor or practice executive determines the staff required to manage the remainder of the day (such as from 1:00 p.m. until closing) and asks for volunteers to go home. If no volunteers emerge, the manager selects staff to send home due to low work volume.

 Part-time staff fill the void and are able to create the "step-up" assistance that is needed.

Part-Time or Per-Diem Staff

Some medical practices keep part-time or per-diem staff on the payroll. They are assigned to work the few sessions when there is high volume. In this fashion, rather than staffing at high levels throughout the week and half-day clinic session, the staffing pattern is changed to respond to peak demand periods. Part-time staff can also assist at the end of the week when the full-time staff may have a long to-do list. Part-time staff fill the void and create the "step-up" assistance that is needed.

Medical Practice Assistants

A medical practice assistant model employs staff with an expanded skill mix to perform each key function in the medical practice.[1] In this model, medical assistants receive expanded training to function

---

[1] The University of Utah is an early proponent of this staffing model. It has fully staffed its outpatient multidisciplinary network with medical practice assistants consistent with its Care by Design program. The replacement of a traditional staffing model with medical practice assistants was budget neutral and added clinical capacity. Personal correspondence with Rob Lloyd, executive director, Ambulatory Services and Community Clinics, University of Utah Health Care, 11/11/10. Also see Magill, Michael K., Robin L. Lloyd, Duane Palmer, Susan A. Terry. 2006. "Successful turnaround of a university-owned, community-based, multidisciplinary practice network." *Ann Fam Med.* 4(Supplement 1):S19–21. www.annfammed.org. Accessed 11/11/2010.

as medical practice assistants (also referred to as clinical associates and other descriptors). They perform an expanded range of work functions to include the traditional work of a medical assistant (such as retrieving and rooming patients and taking vital signs), as well as front office work (managing inbound telephones calls, conducting patient check-in and check-out, and coordinating referrals), and they also function as phlebotomists and imaging technicians. This staffing model replaces the traditional model where medical assistants, receptionists, phlebotomists, and imaging technicians work in specific silos. Instead, "super-trained" medical practice assistants manage each of these roles in an expanded work breadth and scope of responsibility. With this strategy, the staff can be deployed consistent with work fluctuations, rather than be situated in one functional role where they may have idle time or capacity. In some cases, this also permits the staff member to shadow the patient through each step of the patient visit, limiting the handoffs of the patient from one staff member to the next.

The advantages of this model include flexibility to assign staff based on variable work levels, the ability to fully delegate tasks from the physician to the staff, and the ability to recruit and retain high-performing staff who have expanded work variety and are active and contributing members of the care team. The disadvantages of this model are that training is required to ensure that staff can properly manage each of these functions, and accountability for a particular piece of work may be difficult to determine. The latter disadvantage can be overcome by establishing standard work processes. (See Chapter 16, Work Process Redesign, for further information.)

Internal Float Pool

Given the technology in today's medical practices, workers from a temporary employment agency may not have the required access and security to step in to assist the medical practice as they have in the past. Consequently, many medium- to large-sized medical practices are identifying internal float pools of fully trained staff. In the case of the medical practice assistants model previously discussed, the float pool consists of highly trained staff who can seamlessly step in to manage a variety of work functions.[2] Other medical practices hire additional reception staff, schedulers, medical assistants, and nurses and form them into a float pool, based on the medical practice's leave of absence and staff turnover trends. The staff in the float pool are typically the first to be offered a permanent position when it becomes available, as they have knowledge of the medical practice's operations — often from many different vantage points — and can assimilate easily into the culture of the care team.

Multitasking

A more general multitasking model involves an expanded cross-training program so that staff can take on other roles during high peak demand. For example, a medical records technician is trained to conduct patient check-in so this function is staffed appropriately during high patient visit volumes. As another example, a medical assistant is educated regarding inbound telephone calls and scheduling to ensure coverage during peak demand.

The multitasking model involves a more limited approach to cross-training than the medical practice assistants model, yet the additional work assignment for the staff has permanency. For example, on Monday morning the medical assistant rotates to the phones and on Monday afternoon the medical records technician assists with patient check-in. In this fashion, the staff are not merely helping out but, instead, have this as a defined role and responsibility for which they are held accountable.

It is important for staff to understand the entire patient flow process — involving both clinical and business work processes — not just their specific roles and responsibilities. For example, a

---

[2] Personal correspondence with Rob Lloyd, Executive Director, Ambulatory Services and Community Clinics, University of Utah Health Care, 11/11/10.

scheduler who obtains patient demographic and insurance information should be familiar with billing claim forms so that she understands what happens with the information she is asked to collect and verify. Similarly, a check-in staff member who collects time-of-service payments should sit with a biller who is attempting to conduct self-pay account follow-up in order to understand the impact of the work when patients do not pay at the point of care. As a final example, a staff member in the call center should be introduced to the practice suite and shadow the nurse or medical assistant for a period of time to understand their world — and vice versa — so that each can understand the impact of their work on their team member. In this fashion, an integrated care team is developed for the medical practice.

Nurse Leverage

A more recent model that has emerged is the nurse leverage model. In this model, the nurse is trained to take a full history from the patient. The nurse presents the patient to the physician in front of the patient — similar to a resident presenting the patient to the attending faculty physician.[3] (This approach is further described in Chapter 9, Staffing the Visit.)

Volunteers

Community volunteers can serve a number of roles. These include assisting patients during their wait in the reception area, escorting patients to the exam room and to other clinical areas such as laboratory, filing and scanning medical records, and greeting patients upon arrival. Be sure to extend a Health Insurance Portability and Accountability Act (HIPAA) business associates agreement (BAA) to these types of workers to ensure confidentiality and security of patient health information. In many medical practices, volunteers are an important adjunct to the full-time staff.

---

[3] Anderson, Peter, and Marc D. Halley. 2008 "A new approach to making your doctor–nurse team more productive." *Fam Pract Manag.* 15(17):35–40.

STAFFING TO OPTIMIZE FACILITY UTILIZATION

The only revenue-producing spaces in a medical practice are the exam rooms and procedure rooms. If a medical practice can eliminate the sequential process for patient flow, for example, the separate steps of check-in, retrieval, rooming, visit, and check-out, it can reduce the size of its medical practice facility. Rather than ask patients to travel to the work (for example, from the check-in desk to the exam room to the check-out desk), the medical practice can bring the work to the patient in the exam room and eliminate the space needed for these functions—and reduce the queuing and wait time for patients when they visit the medical practice.

Eliminating the Patient Check-In Station

Many medical practices have eliminated the traditional check-in station — and its associated staffing — by performing business preparation for the visit before the visit takes place. The work of verifying information and collecting patient time-of-service payments is conducted in the exam room. If previsit functions have been fully performed, the only activity required at check-in is to verify demographic and insurance information in the event a change has recently occurred, obtain waivers and other signatures, and collect time-of-service payments. Each of these functions can be performed in the exam room by clinical support staff. A number of medical practices have taken this concept further and eliminated the waiting room or reception area altogether, with patients escorted to the exam rooms immediately upon arrival.

Eliminating the Patient Check-Out Station

Other medical practices have eliminated the traditional check-out station — and its associated staffing. This change to the patient flow process and hence to staffing is assisted by an electronic health record. The patient can be reappointed or scheduled for his or her follow-up tests and procedures in the exam room by clinical support staff or scheduling staff.

Eliminating Both Check-In and Check-Out Stations

Still other medical practices have eliminated both the patient check-in and check-out stations altogether. They conduct all clinical and business functions in the exam room, thereby altering their staffing deployment model for the front office.

Either change — eliminating the patient check-in station or eliminating the check-out station (or both) — will alter the patient flow process and, consequently, the staffing model of a medical practice. These changes are consistent with the medical practice assistants model in which staff are trained and capable of handling traditional medical assistant roles, as well as front office and ancillary work functions.

Dual-Shift Schedule

A number of medical practices have extended their patient access hours and improved their facility utilization by running a dual-shift schedule. One set of physicians and support staff work from 7:00 a.m. to 2:00 p.m., for example, with another set working from 2:00 p.m. to 9:00 p.m. Patients love expanded access to care and the per-unit cost of visits for the medical practice is lower. In essence, every medical practice is paying for its space 24/7 but utilizing it only a small fraction of that time. The dual-shift model of care and its associated staffing pattern increases facility utilization, thereby reducing the cost per visit, with the high fixed costs associated with the space spread over more patients.

> The dual-shift model of care and its associated staffing pattern increases facility utilization and spreads the cost over more patients, thereby reducing cost per visit.

WORK SEGMENTATION STRATEGIES

There are times when a medical practice simply cannot afford to hire the number of staff required for the work or is short-staffed for a period of time despite the best planning efforts. There are also times when staff have been delegated a high volume of work tasks and find it hard to prioritize their time to attend to each task. In these situations, consider segmentating staff time to each delegated task to ensure that attention and expertise are paid to the work.

Work Segmentation by Day. For example, a staff member who is tasked with conducting payment posting, insurance account follow-up, and denial management may work under a segmentation strategy to focus energy and attention to each of these tasks. A schedule is developed, and the staff is asked to work on different tasks during different work shifts. For example:

Monday, Tuesday, Wednesday morning:	Account follow-up
Thursday, Friday morning:	Denial management
Monday through Friday afternoon:	Payment posting

Note that the exact work segmentation hours for each task depend on the work volume and complexity. Use the staffing workload ranges previously discussed in this book to identify the amount of time to allocate to each task.

Work Segmentation by Task. Another way to segment work is to delegate it in manageable chunks rather than assigning a full scope of work to a staff member. For example, if a medical practice has a shortage of billing account follow-up staff, it can train a team member to follow up on one specific claim denial only and delegate only those specific accounts to the staff member, training the staff member to a specific, defined work process. In this fashion, a team member can step in to carry out work functions without having the full scope of knowledge of a billing representative. By segmenting the work and training just for that segment, some of the work can be delegated and managed during an unplanned staff shortage.

WORK EXTENSION STRATEGIES

A number of medical practices have decreased their staffing levels by asking current staff to take on added responsibilities. The salary savings from the vacant positions are often used to increase the compensation or provide for a bonus pool for those staff extending their work breadth and scope. The advantages of this approach are many. The best and the brightest staff often can assume added responsibilities and accountability; by paying them additional compensation or bonuses, they can be recognized for this additional work. The staff who are delegated increased responsibility often have a sense of loyalty and engagement with the medical practice above that of a traditional salaried employee. They take ownership in the work and recognize their role as a partner in the practice and as an integral member of the care team.

Examples of work extension strategies include:

> *Medical assistant rooms for two physicians.* One medical assistant rooms patients for two physicians, with one nurse on the phone. In this model, the medical assistant extends his or her scope from one to two physicians. She is on her feet the entire time rooming and anticipating physician needs. In this model, we often have a lag start and end time for the physicians so that the flow of patients throughout the facility can occur in a more streamlined fashion. This model works well with physicians who are fairly self-sufficient based on their practice style and/or their specialty.

> *Nurse extension for quality and safety.* Nurses are asked to take on quality and patient safety projects. Rather than focus this work with one nurse or hire a quality/safety officer, each nurse is delegated a component of quality and safety duties that extends staff knowledge and facilitates their engagement.

➤ *Extended work scope for billing.* A billing representative working insurance account follow-up is asked to extend the scope of his or her work by also managing payment posting and working claim denials. In this fashion, the staff member is able to exercise the full scope of work involved in identifying the reasons for zero payment or under-level payments. Accountability rests fully with this staff member to manage reimbursement from the payers.

WORK ROTATION STRATEGIES

Work rotation strategies are a great way to ensure that staff have the skills and knowledge to perform multiple tasks throughout the practice. Work rotation involves identifying specific days or sessions per day during which the staff member engages in one type of work; other days or sessions are devoted to a different type of work. Examples of work rotation include:

➤ *Nurse flow and telephones.* One nurse is assigned to the telephones and one nurse is involved in patient flow. In the afternoon, these nurses switch roles. Rather than rotate the work by day, another option is to rotate the work by week.

➤ *Manage the queue.* When patients queue up at the front desk, a staff member presses a buzzer or sends a text message to another staff member who arrives at the front desk and opens up another window for check-in. This is similar to a grocery store or bank where more check-out aisles or teller windows open to manage customers in the queue. In this fashion, the additional check-in staff member rotates into the work throughout the day based on workload fluctuation.

➤ *Nurse rotational model.* Nurses rotate specific roles on a weekly basis, such as checking the automated referral line, creating labels for immunizations, and maintaining inventory of supplies and drugs. In this fashion, each nurse is involved in these functions and has a specific work function that supports the team as a whole.

SUMMARY

As we described in this chapter, there are a number of innovative staffing strategies available as you work to align your medical practice with current conditions. The strategies help in aligning staff with the actual work to be performed, replacing the traditional static staffing model. The strategies also help medical practices optimize a key expenditure of the medical practice: the facility in which care is provided. Facility optimization permits medical practices to reduce per-unit healthcare costs. Explore these innovative staffing strategies on a routine basis, particularly prior to filling a vacant position. There may be an opportunity to reassign or delegate work (and potentially prevent the need to hire a new staff member) that permits your current staff to operate more efficiently or become more active members of your care team.

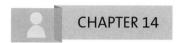

CHAPTER 14

Part-Time Staff and Virtual Staff

There will likely be a "middle ground," a hybrid approach with a smaller office, less commuting, and the flexibility to work where one is most comfortable. That is probably the model that will be adopted by more companies as technology improves, as our economy becomes even more globalized, and as concerns about the environmental impact of commuting grow.

—Max Chafkin
Inc. Magazine Senior Writer
The Case, and the Plan for the Virtual Company

Many corporations have worked to facilitate work–life balance, work-at-home models, and part-time staffing models to attract and retain talent. Healthcare as an industry has lagged somewhat in this area; however, a number of opportunities are available should you elect to transition away from a traditional staffing model of full-time staff physically based at the practice site.

In this chapter, we discuss:

➤ Part-time staff
➤ Virtual staff

PART-TIME STAFF

If your medical practice has high variability in patient visit volume by day of week and session per day, consider part-time staff. There are two distinct strategies: (1) replace full-time staff with part-time staff, and (2) use part-time staff to augment your full-time staff. Medical practices can no longer afford to have numerous employees sitting idle on a particular half-day session or day of the week due to variable provider levels or variable work levels within the practice. When a physician is in surgery or out on a particular half-day session of the week, there is always catch-up work that can be done by the staff in the medical practice. However, more and more medical practices are recognizing that their operating margins are simply too thin to schedule staff when providers are out of the office. This is an excellent opportunity to staff with part-time employees or replace full-time staff with part-time staff.

> With part-time staff on board, the medical practice can achieve productivity gains and also meet patient expectations for service in a way that is difficult for the full-time staff member who is trying to play catch-up at the end of a busy week.

Similarly, when a medical practice has a high volume of patients, such as on Monday afternoon, bringing in a part-time or contract worker for that session of the day can often relieve the considerable workload of the full-time staff so they can start their week in a more planned and focused fashion. This can lead to increases in productivity throughout the week, rather than the full-time staff member going home overly stressed. It can also reduce overtime accumulation; with the part-time staff member supplementing the work of full-time staff, the staff can go home at a regular time or the part-time staff can stay the extended hours.

With part-time staff on board, the medical practice can achieve productivity gains and also meet patient expectations for service in a way that is difficult for the full-time staff member who is trying to play catch-up at the end of a busy week.

Contract workers are increasingly being hired by today's organizations due to their lower cost (health benefit savings) and temporary nature.[1] Contingent or contract workers are typically used to meet seasonal demand or vacation coverage. It is important to ensure that the appropriate business associates agreements are in place to protect patient data (consistent with the Health Insurance Portability and Accountability Act [HIPAA]). It is also important that contract workers have access to and are trained in the technology of the medical practice, for example, the electronic health record or practice management system.

Given today's technological dependence in medical practices, some of the options for temporary agency assistance are limited. Temporary agency workers can answer the telephones, for example, but they may not be able to create an electronic message or have the security access to document in the electronic health record. Thus, medical practices that previously relied on temporary employees are increasingly recognizing the need to develop internal part-time staff or float pools, with staff fully trained in the technology and systems.

Recruitment of Part-Time Staff

Recruit part-time staff using the tools provided in Chapter 18, Grow, Hire, Share, or Outsource. Many markets have well-trained medical practice professionals in their community who welcome the opportunity to work part time. Other sources of part-time staff are described in the following sections.

College students. College students with an interest in healthcare, such as nursing students or pre-med students, can be tapped to work in

---

[1] Davidson, Paul. "Contract workers swelling ranks." *USA Today*. Money Section. Dec. 2, 2009, p. B-1.

> Student interns are another source of part-time staff. These students often have a vested interest in performing well and can be a valuable addition to the care team.

the medical practice on a part-time basis. Some work-study programs will reimburse part of the students' wages for this work.

Student interns. Student interns are another source of part-time staff. They can be paid or unpaid, depending on the program.[2] These students often have a vested interest in performing well in the practice because this experience can launch them in their career and/or help them to complete their study requirements. Many student interns are an exceptional addition to the traditional full-time staff in a medical practice.

The opportunity to have a cadre of per-diem or part-time staff available to the medical practice should be pursued. More than part-timers, many of these staff members are wholeheartedly committed to the practice and its physicians and have long-standing relationships with the medical practice.

> Medical practices that previously relied on temporary agencies are increasingly recognizing the need to develop internal part-time staff or float pools with staff fully trained to the systems and technology.

VIRTUAL STAFF

A number of work functions in a medical practice can be performed remotely. Traditionally referred to as telecommuters, these virtual

---

[2] Oetjen, Reid M., and Dawn M. Oetjen. 2009. "Free labor! How to successfully use student Interns in your practice." *J. Med. Pract. Manage.* 24(6):376–380.

employees can be instrumental to practice success and require no physical work space at the practice site. Advances in technology permit virtual employees to participate in collective forums, such as meetings, while conducting their work from home (or, in actuality, from wherever they have the required access to technology). Witness the many buildings and office locations of staff at some of our largest medical practices. They may be next door or down the street or even across town. The case could be made that if the staff are not involved in face-to-face visits with the patient and do not need to be co-located to perform their job or cover for a colleague, their work can be performed wherever they have access to the tools they need (and the appropriate confidentiality and security of these tools).

> Advances in technology permit virtual employees to participate in collective forums, such as meetings, while conducting their work from home (or, in actuality, from wherever they have the required access to technology).

The types of positions that are suitable for working from a remote site include the following:

Telephone nurse triage staff. With electronic health records, nurses are able to manage inbound patient telephone calls without needing to be in proximity to the medical practice and its physicians. Although co-location of nurses and physicians is often viewed as optimal, the fact is that many physicians are not available to the nurse for in-person communication during the day; much of this interaction is already conducted by telephone or via text messaging.

Care managers. With a list of patients and their pertinent records, care managers can contact patients at home during hours convenient to the patient. The care manager does not need to be physically present in the medical practice to conduct this work.

Health and wellness coaches. Similarly, health and wellness coaches work from flow sheets on their patients or via the electronic health record. They can contact patients by telephone wherever they have access to the technology and confidentiality for patient interaction.

Charge entry staff. Manual charge tickets can be batched and available for charge entry within 24 hours by utilizing telecommuting staff. Similarly, with electronic charge entry, virtual staff are able to review and audit coding and charge entry from a remote location.

Open claims follow-up staff. Access to payer Websites dominates this work function, which can be performed remotely for a medical practice by staff who have access to the technology.

Patient collections staff. Access to the practice management system to view patients' accounts can be made available off-site for customer service representatives to place telephone calls to patients for outstanding account follow-up.

Transcriptionists. As long as the staff member has the appropriate technology, transcription can be conducted off-site. In fact, many healthcare organizations outsource this to other countries.

Whether the staff member is physically based in the medical practice, works in a separate building, or works from home, it is important to identify the tools and oversight that are required for the work functions and to ensure that HIPAA and other security measures are in place to protect patient data.

SUMMARY

In this chapter, we drew attention to the important role that part-time and virtual staff can play in a medical practice as part of the care team. Healthcare as an industry has been late in taking advantage of alternative work arrangements. However, where they do exist, they often work well, with these staff considered active contributors to the care team.

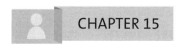

CHAPTER 15

Role Options for Nonphysician Providers

If you are not willing to have midlevel providers work with a high degree of autonomy you are wasting your time and theirs.

—Frank J. Chapman, MBA, COO
Asheville Gastroenterology Associates P.A.

The role of nonphysician providers has changed over time. No longer is the nonphysician provider, such as a nurse practitioner or physician assistant, simply bridging a gap in care delivery or shadowing the physician during the day. Instead, focused roles and responsibilities related to independent practice, combined with expected performance and financial outcomes, have created a more formalized role for these providers in a medical practice.

In this chapter, we:

- ➤ Review the definition and types of nonphysician providers
- ➤ Review the roles nonphysician providers serve in a medical practice
- ➤ Outline the role determination process
- ➤ Provide questions to address in determining role definition
- ➤ Integrate nonphysician providers into the care team
- ➤ Discuss role-dependent compensation plans for nonphysician providers

DEFINITION AND TYPES OF NONPHYSICIAN PROVIDERS

Nonphysician providers (traditionally referred to as midlevel providers or physician extenders) are those caregivers who provide direct hands-on clinical services to patients, for which professional fee billing is typically conducted. Nonphysician providers hold a variety of licensures depending on their specialty. They include nurse practitioners (NPs), physician assistants (PAs), psychologists, social workers, nutritionists, physical therapists, occupational therapists, optometrists, certified registered nurse anesthetists, and midwives. (See the *MGMA Physician Compensation and Production Survey* report for an expanded list of nonphysician providers.)

State laws and regulations dictate the scope and breadth of responsibility of nonphysician providers. In some states, for example, the NP or PA has prescriptive authority; in others they do not. Your medical practice must abide by your state's requirements for nonphysician providers.

Billing for nonphysician providers is complicated, even for experienced practice executives. This involves determining when the billing qualifies as "incident to" the physician's services or if the services need to be billed under the nonphysician provider's name and provider number (Exhibit 15.1). Financial modeling is typically conducted by a medical practice prior to hiring a nonphysician provider to ensure sufficient revenue generation for this expense.

Nonphysician providers are increasingly becoming specialized. For example, in a recent MGMA *Physician Compensation and Production Survey* report, there were 19 subspecialties within the nurse practitioner category and 12 subspecialties reported for physician assistants. These are listed in Exhibit 15.2. It is important to measure and benchmark production and compensation of nonphysician providers at the specialty level, recognizing the specialty-specific nature of their work.

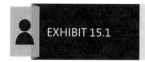

EXHIBIT 15.1

Billing Considerations for Nonphysician Providers

Incident To Billing: The Centers for Medicare & Medicaid Services (CMS) permits your medical practice to receive payment from Medicare for nonphysician services when they are provided "incident to" a physician's services. CMS does not list the billable services that nonphysician providers can perform. Instead, it defers to each state's rules regarding the scope of practice and certification or licensure for those providers.

CMS has specific qualifications to permit the work of nonphysician providers to be billed incident to the physician. For example, CMS states that they must be "services or supplies [that] are furnished as an integral, although incidental, part of the physician's personal professional services in the course of diagnosis or treatment of an injury or illness." Further, the agency asserts that "such a service or supply could be considered incident to when furnished during a course of treatment where the physician performs an initial service and subsequent services of a frequency which reflect his/her active participation in the management of the course of treatment." In addition, CMS indicates that the incident to rules are "limited to situations in which there is direct physician supervision of auxiliary personnel." It further clarifies that "the physician must be present in the office suite and immediately available to provide assistance and direction throughout the time the aide is performing services." A number of other additional requirements for incident to billing should be understood. They are reported at www.cms.gov.

Billing Under the Nonphysician Provider's Name: If the services provided by the nonphysician provider do not qualify for incident to billing, the services must be billed under the nonphysician's name and provider number. The CMS reimbursement rate for nonphysician providers who bill directly is 85 percent of the physician fee schedule. Again, the nonphysician provider must be operating within the scope of the state's requirements for that profession and, in addition, must be in compliance with each payer's rules related to nonphysician provider care.

Source: Elizabeth W. Woodcock, MBA, FACMPE, CPC. Personal communication with author. Used with permission.

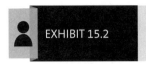

Nurse Practitioner	Physician Assistant
Acute care	Physician Assistant: Surgical
Adult	➢ Cardiothoracic surgery
Cardiology	➢ Orthopaedic
Emergency	Physician Assistant: Primary Care
Endocrinology	➢ Family practice with obstetrics
Family practice with obstetrics	➢ Family practice without obstetrics
Family practice without obstetrics	➢ Internal medicine
Gastroenterology	➢ Pediatric
Gerontology/elder health	➢ Urgent care
Hematology/oncology	Physician Assistant: Nonsurgical/ Nonprimary Care
Internal medicine	➢ Cardiology
Neonatal/perinatal	➢ Dermatology
Neurology	➢ Hospital
Pediatric/child health	➢ Neurology
Psychiatry	➢ Orthopaedic
OB/GYN/women's health	
Nurse practitioner, nonsurgical/ nonprimary care	
Nurse practitioner, primary care	
Nurse practitioner, surgical	

Source: Medical Group Management Association. 2010. *Physician Compensation and Production Survey: 2010 Report Based on 2009 Data*. Englewood, Colo.: Medical Group Management Association. Reprinted with permission.

ROLES OF NONPHYSICIAN PROVIDERS

There are two primary roles nonphysician providers serve in a medical practice: leverage and production. Within the production category, there are four models: full production, limited production, quick-access production, and rotational production.

> There are two primary roles nonphysician providers play in a medical practice: leverage and production.

Leverage Role

Examples of leverage models for the nonphysician provider include:

Care support. Some medical practices employ nonphysician providers to leverage physicians by performing certain work that frees up the physician to see more patients and thereby grow market share. For example, nonphysician providers may review laboratory results, return patient calls, and staff hospital wards.

Care delivery. Further leveraging the physician, nonphysician providers may support care delivery in hospital work and other labor-intensive clinical functions that require provider-specific knowledge (beyond the knowledge and skills of licensed nursing staff).

Continuity of care. In some cases, the PA or NP will be asked to work alongside the physician, or to shadow the physician while the physician is in surgery, making rounds, performing consultations, or in the office setting. "In these instances, the key is to ensure that the nonphysician provider exercises medical decision-making skills at a provider level is not simply functioning as 'buddy.'"[1]

When nonphysician providers are deployed in a leverage model, we expect physicians to have higher clinical production or engage in

---

[1] Frank J. Chapman, MBA, chief operating officer, Asheville Gastroenterology Associates, PA, coined the term PA or NP "buddies" when the nonphysician provider is not fully deployed in a leverage or production model.

expanded clinical activity.[2] By displacing the physician to do other things, the nonphysician provider should be truly leveraging the physician. The compensation paid to nonphysician providers is significant. For NP and PA nonphysician providers, for example, the median annual salary typically ranges from $80,000 to $90,000 (excluding benefits and operating expense). If the nonphysician is not able to truly leverage the physician, a leverage model is likely not financially sustainable for the long term.

Production Role

Many medical practices have replaced the leverage model with a true production model for the nonphysician provider. When nonphysician providers are employed for production purposes, they generally are assigned to one of the following four production types (Exhibit 15.3):

- Full production
- Limited production
- Quick-access production
- Rotational production

If the role of the nonphysician provider on the care team is one of production, the infrastructure and support to the nonphysician provider needs to be similar to that of a physician. This means that nonphysician providers should not be rooming their own patients, managing their own telephone calls, and doing everything themselves, but should be supported by the staff in a medical practice at a level consistent with that provided to physicians.

Full Production Model

In a full production model, nonphysician providers are generally expected to see patient volumes ranging from 65 percent to 100 percent

---

[2] In these instances, it is also important to determine if this type of work can be conducted by licensed clinical support staff, rather than a nonphysician provider.

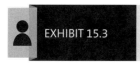

Type of Production Model	Description
Full production	The nonphysician provider is expected to see a high volume of patients, similar to a physician in that specialty.
Limited production	The nonphysician provider is expected to perform a limited scope of patient care activities. For example, the NP or PA may be involved in procedures, surgical assists, and/or treating a specific diagnosis or managing a specific chief complaint.
Quick-access production	The nonphysician provider is expected to see same-day, urgent patients who call or present to the clinic for care.
Rotational production	The physician and nonphysician provider rotate visits with the patient, thereby extending a limited physician resource to expand access to care.

of physicians, provided they are given the infrastructure and support for this productivity in the form of exam rooms and clinical support staff.[3] In some cases, the nonphysician provider is scheduled for clinic on the same day as the physician to whom he or she is assigned

---

[3] The expectation for 65 to 100 percent of clinical production for nonphysician providers has typically been based on primary care models, specifically family practice groups. This is supported by MGMA median data. For example, an NP in family practice without obstetrics reports a median of 3,300 work relative value units (WRVUs), with a physician in the same specialty reporting 4,845 WRVUs (see the MGMA's *Physician Compensation and Production Survey: 2010 Report Based on 2009 Data*). Production expectations for nonphysician providers are based on the role and specialty, with more comparative data available based on nonphysician provider subspecialty.

to permit oversight by the physician (if required by the state or per the physician mentor or supervisor). The scope of practice, level of supervision, and opportunity to generate professional fees for services depends on the state laws and regulations governing nonphysician scope of practice and autonomy, payer requirements, and billing practices. Based on a recent MGMA survey, 46 percent of the better-performing practices that engaged nonphysician providers in their practice reported that the nonphysician provider was in a full production model and was assigned his or her own patient base.[4]

Limited Production Model

In a limited production model, nonphysician providers serve in specialty-specific roles or are devoted to a specific role or patient type. Examples include:

- Conduct procedures

- Serve as surgical assistants

- Gather patient history and conduct work-up

- Provide complex care coordination

- Provide continuity of care in the inpatient setting (thereby reducing length of stay, minimizing repeat tests, and reducing cost of care)

- Provide a specific skill set that may be missing or scarce (for example, see patients with depression or perform well-woman examinations)

- Treat a particular type of patient, for example, those who need physical therapy, speech therapy, nutrition counseling, psychological counseling, or other similar services

These types of production models for nonphysician providers are more limited or focused in scope than those of a full production

---

[4] Medical Group Management Association. 2009. "Practices and Procedures Survey Results, Patient Care Systems" in: *Performance and Practices of Successful Medical Groups: 2009 Report Based on 2008 Data*. Englewood, Colo: Medical Group Management Association; p. 124.

model. This is not to imply that the providers are not fully productive in the course of their care and treatment, but rather to distinguish a provider with a limited focus from one who is essentially
expected to have a patient base similar to that of a physician (the
latter considered a full production model).

Quick-Access Production Model

In some cases, nonphysician providers see a higher volume of
patients than a physician. This can occur when the nonphysician
provider is delegated the same-day, urgent patients who require less
time and intensity than new patients or more complicated patients.
Assigning nonphysician providers to quick-access work can involve
many forms. For example:

> Some medical practices schedule quick-access appointments
  from 7:00 a.m. to 9:00 a.m. or in the evening from 5:00 p.m.
  to 7:00 p.m. Nonphysician providers staff these sessions to
  manage same-day, urgent care visits.

> Some medical practices reserve specific slots during the day
  for urgent care visits on the physician schedule. When the
  physician's schedule is full, the nonphysician provider manages the overflow of same-day, urgent care visits.

> Some medical practices provide advanced access. In these
  models, patients can be seen when they want to be seen by
  their own physician. However, if that physician is out of the
  office, nonphysician providers see and treat the patients who
  require quick access.

> Some medical practices have urgent care clinics held sepa-
  rately from physician office hours. Nonphysician providers
  are asked to staff the urgent care areas, referring more complicated patients to the physicians as medically necessary.

> Some medical practices schedule weekend hours. Nonphysi-
  cian providers work in conjunction with a physician or manage these weekend office hours in a more independent fashion. Note that this is similar to a retail clinic–type of practice

where a nurse practitioner may work in the local drugstore or superstore to see patients who present with certain, defined conditions.

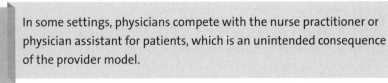

In some settings, physicians compete with the nurse practitioner or physician assistant for patients, which is an unintended consequence of the provider model.

It is important that medical practices understand the consequences of using nonphysician providers in a quick-access production model. If physicians in the medical practice receive compensation based on production, the reassignment of same-day, urgent, or quick-check appointments to nonphysician providers can negatively impact the physician's compensation level. For example, in primary care practices where Evaluation and Management codes are typically billed, this can often pose a problem. If the physician sees the more complex patients who require extra time (thereby seeing a reduced patient visit volume), he or she may not be able to generate the same level of revenue than when seeing a combination of patient visit types, for example, long visits (involving new or complex patients) and short visits (involving routine visits for established patients or quick-check appointments based on a single chief complaint). In some settings, physicians actually compete with the NP or PA for patients, which is an unintended consequence of the model that has been embraced by the medical practice, and an unhealthy relationship between physicians and nonphysician providers may ensue.

Rotational Production Model

Increasingly, nonphysician providers are being used to truly extend a limited physician resource. With a shortage of physicians in many markets, a rotational model involving the physician and nonphysician provider is prevalent. For example, when there is a shortage of medical oncologists in a community, the physician will typically see the patient at the initial visit and then at the patient's third or fourth visit; the patient sees the nonphysician provider at each of the interim visits. Similarly, in primary care or pediatrics, a shortage of physicians leads to a rotational model to expand patient access to care. Many of today's medical specialists have either assimilated or are planning to assimilate nonphysician providers in these types of roles, recognizing the need to expand patient access, given the fact that physicians are becoming a scarce or limited resource.

> With a shortage of physicians in many markets, a rotational model involving the physician and nonphysician provider is prevalent.

ROLE DETERMINATION PROCESS

No one model for the use of nonphysician providers in the medical practice has been embraced as a best practice. Rather, each medical practice should approach its decision based on a number of local and specific challenges. These include, but are not limited to:

- State laws and regulations governing scope of practice, supervision, and billing
- Level of delegation by physicians to nonphysicians
- Current types of patients and patient conditions
- Current patient volumes and patient access challenges
- Current physician and nonphysician provider levels
- Financial position of the medical practice (nonphysician providers are typically paid less than physicians)
- Philosophy regarding the use of nonphysician providers
- Market and patient acceptance of nonphysician providers
- Degree of integration of the care team physicians, nonphysician providers, fellows, residents, nurses, and others
- Focused strategic goals, for example, grow market share or build research programs

➤ Outreach programs, for example, coverage needed at rural health, outreach sites

➤ Continuity of care for complex patients or chronic care patients

➤ Specific patient needs based on volumes, for example, senior patients with durable medical equipment requests, assisted living, family liaison issues, and complex care coordination, or complex patients with extensive care needs

Regardless of the role that is selected for the nonphysician provider in your medical practice, studies have shown that there is an advantage to integrating the nonphysician provider in the care team by standardizing physician collaborations with these providers in a medical practice. Evidence suggests that this standardization helps control costs and increases practice efficiency.[5]

Just as there is no one "right" role for nonphysician providers in a medical practice, there is no "right" volume of nonphysician providers in a medical practice. The volume depends on the role, the size of the medical group, the number of patients, and a host of other similar factors. To analyze the current volume of nonphysician providers and to build the volume based on the work, the staffing strategies discussed in Chapter 4, The Staff Benchmarking Process, and Chapter 5, The Staff Workload Evaluation Process, can be applied.

Typically, when physicians in the medical practice are highly productive and are not able to meet patient access demand, the discussion of whether or not to hire an additional physician for the medical practice begins. If your medical practice reaches this point, revisit your physician and nonphysician provider model and determine whether a different model, an expansion of the current model, or an introduction of a nonphysician provider in the practice makes

---

[5] Anderson, Benjamin, and John Rozich. 2001. "Your practice's most important 'work-in': Bringing certified nurse practitioners on to the treatment team." *MGMA Connexion.* 1(1):6–65.

financial and strategic sense for your practice. The key is to ensure that the nonphysician provider has a full complement of work for the role that your medical practice has identified.

QUESTIONS TO ADDRESS IN ASSESSING ROLE DEFINITION

In many medical practices, it is evident that the nonphysician provider model has evolved over time rather than being formed with a clear and distinct strategy. When a proactive approach toward identifying the specific roles, responsibilities, and goals of the nonphysician provider is used, the outcomes for the nonphysician provider can be measured and then compared with the intended goal.

Questions to be asked and answered regarding the role of the nonphysician provider are provided below to assist in determining whether your provider model has met the intended goal of the medical practice. These questions should be revisited at regular intervals to determine if the nonphysician provider has been deployed consistent with the goals and is having the intended impact on the medical practice. In addition, there may be changes in the medical practice due to market or other factors that warrant a reconsideration of the nonphysician model adopted for your medical practice.

➤ Are nonphysician providers expected to leverage physicians to grow market share? If so, has this strategy been realized or does the medical practice have a relatively flat patient base?

➤ Have the roles and responsibilities been aligned in a care team model, with delegation consistent with the licensure and scope of practice of each of these team members? If that is the goal, has it been realized?

➤ Are nonphysician providers working a distinctly defined role or are they simply bridging the gap and now performing nursing duties that can be further delegated to clinical support staff?

➤ Were nonphysician providers hired to leverage physicians during their clinical time, permitting them to see more patients? If so, has this goal been realized? Are physicians actually seeing larger clinical volumes as this leverage strategy would suggest?

➤ Were nonphysician providers hired to perform care coordinating functions due to the part-time nature of physicians or faculty or due to type and severity of patient illness? If so, has this been achieved, or are nonphysician providers involved in work that is more appropriately conducted by clinical support staff, for example, scheduling tests and procedures or following up on lab and test results?

> In many medical practices, it is evident that the nonphysician provider model has evolved over time rather than being formed with a clear and distinct strategy.

INTEGRATING NONPHYSICIAN PROVIDERS INTO THE CARE TEAM

Beyond the specific role identified for your nonphysician providers, there should be no turf issues between the nonphysician providers and nurses, nonphysician providers and fellows or residents, and nonphysician providers and physicians. In addition, each member of the care team should work to educate patients on the integration of nonphysician providers and the important role they play in the medical practice. This can include practice brochures outlining the role of the nonphysician provider in the medical practice and one-on-one discussions with patients regarding next steps and the role of nonphysician providers in the care and treatment plan. As we noted earlier, it is important to provide the same level of infrastructure and support to the nonphysician provider that is extended to the phy-

sician if the intent is a full production model. This includes staff allocated to support patient flow, nurse triage, and scheduling, as well as
an appropriate number of exam rooms.

Despite embracing nonphysician providers in the care team,
philosophical differences regarding their role in a medical practice
may emerge. For example, should each physician be required to
use the nonphysician provider? Should letters be sent to referring
physicians over the signature of a nonphysician provider? Should
nonphysician providers be on consult services or take first call, or
should these activities be more appropriately staffed by a physician
(or, in the case of an academic practice, by a faculty member, fellow, or resident)? These and similar challenges need to be resolved
in a medical practice if the intent is to fully realize a well-coordinated physician and nonphysician provider group practice.

The keys to effectively integrating nonphysician providers into the
care team are to:

- Define the goal or expected outcome of nonphysician
  providers
- Define their specific roles on the care team
- Define specific performance expectations related to work quality and quantity
- Determine appropriate funding sources and compensation
  consistent with their work

Impact of Nonphysician Providers on the Medical Practice

MGMA publishes an annual survey report devoted specifically to
data from better-performing medical practices. The report, *Performance and Practices of Successful Medical Groups,* presents data and
case studies of medical practices that have performed better than

their peers in terms of financial and other measures. In a recent survey, better-performing practices were asked to identify the impact of nonphysician providers in their practice. The results of the survey are reported in Exhibit 15.4. The top three advantages of having nonphysician providers included the ability to accommodate patient demand, increased physician productivity, and enhanced revenue for the medical practice.

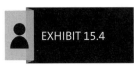

| EXHIBIT 15.4 | Impact of Nonphysician Providers in the Medical Practice |

Effect	Percentage
Accommodated patient demand	60.27%
Increased physician productivity	57.26%
Enhanced revenue	52.88%
Increased patient satisfaction	48.77%
Increased patient base	35.89%
Added ancillary services	18.90%
Improved patient safety	14.79%

Source: Medical Group Management Association. 2009. "Practices and Procedures Survey Results, Human Resource Management" in *Performance and Practices of Successful Medical Groups: 2009 Report Based on 2008 Data*. Englewood, Colo: Medical Group Management Association; p. 120.

In addition to the above findings, the survey also indicates that 4.93 percent of better performers reported no revenue gain or loss associated with nonphysician providers and 1.64 percent reported reduced revenue as an effect of nonphysician providers. Reprinted with permission.

COMPENSATION FOR NONPHYSICIAN PROVIDERS

There are a number of books and articles devoted to compensation plans for nonphysician providers.[6] This book does not aim to address the topic in depth. However, it is important to raise awareness that it may be appropriate to use a different compensation plan depending on the role the nonphysician provider plays in the medical practice. There is no one-size-fits-all when it comes to compensation plans and the nonphysician provider.

Revenue Treatment

Many medical practices pay a flat salary to the nonphysician provider for a two-year period, during which the provider is also eligible for incentives if net collections exceed the salary (and benefit) amount. In these situations, the nonphysician provider may, for example, receive 10 percent of net collections generated greater than compensation in year one and 25 percent of net collections greater than compensation in year two. If the nonphysician provider is deployed in a production model, after the initial two-year period, he or she may be on an "eat what you kill" formula, essentially required to generate revenue to cover his or her cost of practice, salary, and benefits.

This compensation plan, however, may not be appropriate when the nonphysician provider is employed in a leverage model or a limited production model. For example, if the nonphysician provider has been asked to leverage the physician or provide continuity of care to patients, the nonphysician provider typically cannot generate revenue at the level of his or her full production counterparts. This is due, in part, to billing and reimbursement requirements by payers and, in part, to the type of work the nonphysician provider has been

---

[6] See Johnson, Bruce, and Deborah Walker Keegan. 2006. *Physician Compensation Plans: State-of-the-Art Strategies*. Englewood, Colo.: Medical Group Management Association.

tasked to perform. Thus, nonphysician providers who are in leverage or limited production models are often placed on a base plus incentive compensation model.

As these two examples illustrate, a compensation model that is role dependent is required for the nonphysician provider. We recommend that a medical practice first identify the specific roles the nonphysician provider is to play and then determine the appropriate compensation plan to recognize and reward this work and effort.

Expense Treatment

In physician-owned medical practices, when nonphysician providers are employed to leverage physicians, thereby permitting physicians to increase production, the cost of the nonphysician provider is typically assigned as a direct expense to the physician who benefits from the support. If the nonphysician provider is serving a role that assists the hospital or for which the physician is not receiving direct production credit, then the nonphysician provider is often paid by another source, for example, the medical practice or hospital.

In the academic practice setting, nonphysician providers are typically funded via a combination of hospital, departmental, and grant funding, depending on the role of the nonphysician provider. If a nonphysician provider is staffing an inpatient hospital service, that position is typically funded by the hospital. If the hospital is not willing or able to fund the position, then the academic department is placed in the difficult position of determining whether it needs to alter or discontinue services, given its other priorities and commitments.

SUMMARY

In this chapter, we discussed the role options for nonphysician providers and the importance of ensuring that the initial goals for them have been met. When appropriately deployed and supported, nonphysician providers play a valuable role in leveraging physician clinical time, increasing clinical production and patient access, providing continuity of care, managing complex care coordination, and performing specialty-specific roles as integral members of the care team.

PART 5

Process Improvement

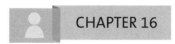

CHAPTER 16

Work Process Redesign

What you cannot and should never promise is that no one's job will change. As people redesign processes, it means changing the way they work.

—Mastering Patient Flow: Using Lean Thinking
to Improve Your Patient Operations, 3rd Edition

The staffing deployment model of a medical practice is dependent on the work volume and the work processes that the staff have been tasked to perform. Some of the work processes in today's medical practices are highly encumbered and involve multiple steps, hand-offs of work from one staff member to another, rework, checking of work, and other similar waste that has an impact on staff efficiency and, consequently, the number of staff needed in a medical practice. The key to work process redesign is to balance staff autonomy and self-management with standard work and expectations.

In this chapter, we discuss:

- ➤ Lean management systems and principles
- ➤ Standard and disciplined work
- ➤ Streamlined work processes

LEAN MANAGEMENT SYSTEMS AND PRINCIPLES

"Lean" is a formal management system that originated in Japan. A number of integrated delivery systems and medical practices have adopted lean principles to galvanize their physicians and staff to improve work processes to minimize waste — wasted time, materials, people, and processes — and to focus on improving value to patients.[1] Lean tools provide a common language and vocabulary and a consistent approach toward identification of waste and non–value-added processes. Lean tools include rapid process improvement workshops; value-stream maps (a form of process flowcharts); quality improvement tools such as brainstorming, cause-and-effect diagrams, and affinity diagrams; standardized measures; visual displays of process steps; and transparent performance outcomes.

The goals of lean are to focus the energies of the medical practice on reducing waste (including wasted time, defects, errors, and nonvalue-added work steps and processes) and continually improving work processes. Many medical practices have piled on more and more work but have not taken any work away. The time has not been taken to redesign work processes in support of the physician or the patient. Instead, physicians and staff are asked to work harder and faster, and patients are asked to overlook or engage in encumbered processes. This approach is self-limiting.

Lean, when adopted as a formal management system, must be led by the top leaders in the organization. In fact, many organizations' leaders travel to Japan to learn the lean methods and tools first-hand. However, lean adopted as a philosophy and tool can be used by anyone to improve work processes. In this section, we focus on the concept of lean as a tool to reduce the complexity and encumbered nature of work processes assigned to the staff and streamline the work, with a focus on doing the right things and doing them right.

---

[1] Examples of healthcare organizations that have embraced "lean" are Group Health of Puget Sound, Virginia Mason Medical Center, and Park Nicollet Health Services. More information on lean is provided in the Additional Resources Section.

Lean serves as a galvanizing force to overcome inertia to change, and it serves as a catalyst to create a new organizational culture.

To get started with lean, a medical practice needs to become familiar with lean management and the tools involved in process improvement, such as flowchart mapping, measurement tools, visual cues (such as labels and white boards to see process flow), and continuous quality improvement tools such as Plan-Do-Check-Act (PDCA). Resources for lean and continuous quality improvement are provided in the Appendix.

A nine-step framework for value-stream mapping and process improvement is presented in Exhibit 16.1. The nine steps generally summarize the processes involved in lean and continuous process improvement. This is not intended to be a formal guide to lean; rather it is intended to provide a brief overview of the work involved in analyzing and redesigning a work process and the tools that will typically help along this journey.

When lean is adopted as a management system for a medical practice, physicians and staff are trained on how to use the tools and methods. As a consequence, some of the steps can be short-circuited. Rapid process improvement teams are indeed rapid (often completing their charter within three days); a pilot is conducted swiftly and the expectation is that the pilot will indeed be spread throughout the organization. There are executive leaders and sponsors for the work, and process owners and teams are focused on improving the value stream for the patient. Over time, lean becomes the way the medical practice does business. Thus, it serves as a galvanizing force to overcome inertia to change and it serves as a catalyst to create a new organizational culture.

An example of a traditional work process used in a medical practice is provided in Exhibit 16.2. It depicts a basic flowchart of the process

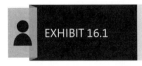

| EXHIBIT 16.1 | Nine-Step Framework for Process Redesign |

Step 1 Select a process for redesign
Purpose: To identify a process in the patient value stream that is currently encumbered or not adding value to the patient

Step 2 Identify a rapid process improvement team
Purpose: To identify project sponsors and team members and identify operating agreement, team charge, and timeline

Step 3 Identify customer and patient needs and wants
Purpose: To identify the value-added steps important to the customer

Step 4 Map the existing process
Purpose: To gain an understanding of the current state, the what, and the why to ensure understanding of the work process to be redesigned

Step 5 Measure process performance
Purpose: To gain the needed performance understanding of the targeted process through the collection of appropriate and relevant data (for example, data that add clarity to the process parameters) and to translate the data into redesign goals (for example, level of improvement, time, cost)

Step 6 Redesign the existing process and create value stream map
Purpose: To redesign the current process to reduce waste and improve value

Step 7 Pilot the redesigned process
Purpose: To pilot the redesign and make changes as needed consistent with a PDCA process

Step 8 Develop implementation plan
Purpose: To develop the organization-wide implementation plan

Step 9 Implement the redesign
Purpose: To spread the redesign throughout the organization

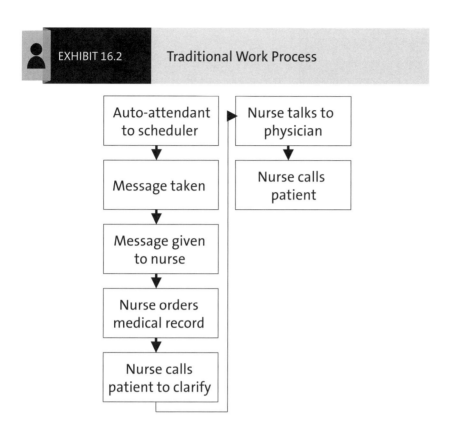

EXHIBIT 16.2   Traditional Work Process

Note: Flowchart does not include repeat calls or telephone tag.

used for a same-day appointment request from a patient. The shape of a rectangle indicates each discrete step in the work process, and the arrows show the sequence of the steps. In this flowchart, the process starts when the patient calls the medical practice and listens to the auto-attendant function, selecting the option to schedule an appointment. The process ends when the nurse places a telephone call to the patient to notify him or her as to whether the same-day request for an appointment has been granted. This flowchart reflects the process prior to conducting process redesign to reduce waste and improve value-added steps to the patient.

Exhibit 16.3 depicts the newly redesigned process, a considerable improvement over the previous one. There are only two steps to

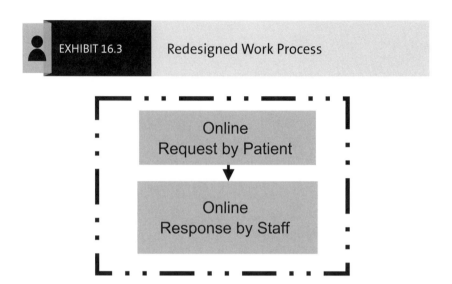

EXHIBIT 16.3   Redesigned Work Process

the process. Step 1 is the patient using the Web portal to submit an online request for a same-day appointment, and step 2 is the online response by a staff member assigned to manage the Web portal. As this diagram demonstrates, the number of steps in the process and the cycle time for the process are dramatically reduced. The process is redesigned to reduce waste and focus on the value-added steps through a patient lens.

This is just one example of the many processes that are ripe for lean principles and quality improvement tools to enhance value and reduce unnecessary work variation and waste. By streamlining the work assigned to staff, a staffing model can be adopted that improves staff efficiency and effectiveness in service to patients and that matches the staff to the work. Highly encumbered work processes not only dissatisfy patients, but also require more staff than processes that have been redesigned using lean tools and techniques.

STANDARD AND DISCIPLINED WORK

When work is fully defined, a flowchart and standardized steps outline the processes and tools the staff are to use in the course of their work. Though it may look as if the intellectual capital and creativity of the staff are minimized by creating standard work, this is not what is intended. Instead, by standardizing certain processes to ensure staff are working in a systematic fashion, time is freed up for them to focus on creativity and innovation in order to improve their work and their work environment. Thus, standard work is not synonymous with a robotic approach to the work. Instead, picture it as a way to get work accomplished in an efficient and systematic fashion so that innovation and creativity can emerge.

> In a typical day, we experience "time creep." Time simply flies by, and it is very difficult to ensure that all the required functions and tasks are attended to.

In a medical practice, there is a lot of work to do each and every day. The time to complete a specific function will take about as long as the staff member has time to complete it. Everyone seems busy, and everyone believes he or she is busy. But at the end of the day, when asked, many staff and managers are not able to relate their accomplishments. The day was confused with a lot of patients and tasks and paper. But what truly was accomplished to move the organization forward? In a typical day, we experience "time creep." Time simply flies by, and it is very difficult to ensure that all the required functions and tasks are attended to. Often the work that needs to be performed by a medical practice is in the hearts and minds of the people. And although the people have good intentions, the day can go by without key work processes being performed, with the work becoming hit-and-miss. The adoption of standard work provides the intentional discipline needed to ensure that key tasks are performed each day, every day, and that they are not overlooked due to the exigencies of the practice. This work becomes ingrained and becomes a system property.

An Example of Standard Work

Picture a medical practice with 20 practice sites.[2] Every day at 8:00 a.m. a huddle occurs at each of the sites. The work that is conducted in the huddle is standardized—the same questions are asked each and every time. The adoption of standard work permits this orchestrated approach to occur. If not, only those medical practices with a strong and determined leader will even hold the huddle. If not, those physicians and staff who want the huddle will not be able to make it happen, and key information is therefore not shared with the care team.

Policies and procedures are important elements of standard work, but more important are the time and manner in which the work is conducted. For example, let's suppose you have a policy to conduct huddles each morning and each afternoon. That's great. It is one of the communication methods we strongly recommend to make sure that everyone is on the same page and ready for the patients who are presenting for care. This is the time that the physician helps the scheduler recognize that she or he is double-booked, for example, with two patients who have a history of depression. By evaluating the schedule in a huddle, the team can direct staff to reschedule one of the patients.

This all sounds well and good. However, how many medical practices have missed their huddle? How many huddles have been held that did not review the key agenda items intended? It is so easy in a medical practice for the daily operations of the practice to take over and for the intended work functions to get skipped or covered in a less-than-optimal manner.

> By expecting the huddle to be held and the formal agenda to be followed, medical practice leaders ensure that the work will be performed in a standard, systematic, and efficient manner—each time, every time.

[2] The author wishes to acknowledge Group Health of Puget Sound for its groundbreaking work in using lean management to create standard work.

For standard work to occur with a huddle, create specific expectations, ensure that everyone in the practice is aware of the expectations, and ensure the work is actually performed through the use of management rounds and by keeping a visual display that shows that the work was performed. Continuing with our huddle example: At 8:00 a.m. and at 1:00 p.m. staff hold a five-minute huddle. The physician, nurse, medical assistant, and scheduler participate in the huddle.[3] The agenda is standardized as follows:

➤ Which patients are scheduled to come in this morning (or afternoon)?

➤ What preparation has been conducted and what preparation is still needed for the visit?

➤ What worked in the last clinic session and what didn't?

➤ What can we do differently as a team to make it work?

➤ Let's review one operational improvement process that we have adopted.

By expecting the huddle to be held and the formal agenda to be followed and by creating a transparent display that records that the huddle was indeed held, the practice performs the work in a standard, systematic, and efficient fashion. In addition, everyone knows the questions in advance; a comment that a particular process is not working, for example, is immediate feedback to the team to improve. Similarly, a comment that a process worked particularly well is immediate positive feedback that the team is in sync.

As we discussed in Chapter 11, Staffing for Medical Records and Electronic Health Records, with the introduction of electronic health records, standard work and an expanded work scope are required for clinical support staff. This is important, not only to ensure the appropriate infrastructure for the patient visit and for virtual medicine, but also to ensure that the meaningful use criteria for electronic health records are consistently met.

---

[3] Some medical practices include other members of the team in the huddle, such as the on-site biller, check-in/check-out staff, laboratory technician, and imaging technician.

Many organizations are striving to redefine the work scope of their staff to provide work that is challenging and meaningful, while simultaneously creating standard work. An industry other than healthcare that is working to be lean is reported in Exhibit 16.4. As this exhibit demonstrates, by expanding the scope of work and making it more challenging and diverse, as well as expecting standard work, accountability increases.

By defining standard work, everyone knows precisely what is expected and the medical practice becomes more systematic and purposeful in its work.

Additional examples of standard work in the medical practice are provided in Exhibit 16.5. The "who," "how," and "when" the work is to be performed are spelled out and checklists are used as a tool to help physicians and staff make sure that each of these standard work elements is performed. Recent studies have shown the valuable use of checklists in operating rooms to reduce variability and to ensure standard work takes place. Checklists provided to physicians and staff in the medical practice can ensure that the medical practice, too, is reducing variability and performing standard and consistent work — each time, every time.

Standard work goes beyond that which is typically found in a standard policy and procedure manual. Everyone is expected to do the same work and perform the same process steps, with the same timelines. Importantly, this is done each time, every time. The goal is to reduce unwanted variation in the work and ensure a standard experience by the patient that is focused on the value-added steps needed to treat and care for the patient.

> Everyone is expected to do the same work and perform the same process steps, with the same timelines. Importantly, this is done each time, every time.

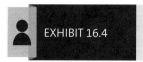

EXHIBIT 16.4   Standard Work at the Golf Course

Professionals manage golf courses. The day-to-day work involved in maintaining a golf course typically rests with staff who perform standard work. This is how one golf course handles the process.

> ➤ There are five groundskeepers assigned to maintain the course.

> ➤ Rather than assign each groundskeeper a specific task, such as edging or mowing, each worker is assigned to specific holes and is held accountable for all of the maintenance required for those holes.

> ➤ Each worker is given color-coded equipment. For example, one staff has a cart with equipment that is red, his colleague has yellow equipment, and so on. In this fashion, the staff member is responsible for his or her own equipment (reducing the amount of lost and borrowed equipment that occurred in the past).

> ➤ Each day the staff are expected to perform similar assignments. For example, they are expected to roll the greens in a specific direction on one day, edge the holes on another day, and so on.

The groundskeeping staff thus have been given more challenging and diverse work. In addition, they are expected to perform standard work, yet they are largely self-managed during the day. The elegance of this approach also permits accountability. Since the staff are assigned to specific holes, it is readily apparent who is performing well and who may need assistance or improvement. In addition, course managers can visually see the status of each staff member's work, as the color-coded equipment makes the staff highly visible when they are out on the course.

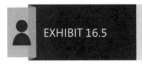

EXHIBIT 16.5

Examples of Standard Work
in the Medical Practice

Chart Documentation

➤ The visit notes are documented during the visit by the physician when feasible, however, no later than noon for morning appointments and end of day for afternoon appointments.

➤ The visit notes are to follow the standard for completeness established by the medical practice.

Charge Tickets

➤ The charge ticket is completed by the physician the same day the patient is seen.

➤ The physician determines the procedure and diagnosis codes for billing purposes and orders the codes.

➤ The physician reports the laboratory and tests that were ordered and any supplies that were used.

➤ The nurse reviews the charge ticket for accuracy and completeness.

➤ The nurse checks six areas on the charge ticket: procedure code, diagnosis code, supplies, medications, injections, and physician signature.

➤ The charge ticket is reviewed and checked by the nurse on the day the patient is seen.

➤ The billing staff review the charge ticket and affix appropriate modifiers the day they are received.

➤ The billing staff identify any missing information and communicate this to the physician on the day received.

➤ The physician responds with updated and complete information within 24 hours.

(Continued on next page)

Test Results Reporting

> The nurse reviews the results; all abnormal results are brought to the attention of the physician through the in-box marked "urgent."

> The nurse reviews abnormal results with the physician by end of day and places calls to the patient the same day.

> A letter is sent to the patient to inform the patient of normal results; a copy of the full results report mailed to the patient within 24 hours of receipt.

Rooming the Patient

> The medical assistant introduces herself to the patient with a standard greeting, for example, "Hello, I'm Sally. I am Dr. Green's medical assistant and I will be assisting with your visit today."

> The medical assistant reviews the reason for the patient's visit.

> The medical assistant takes the patient's height, weight, blood pressure, and temperature.

> The medical assistant reviews the current list of medications, updates it, and determines if prescription renewals are needed.

> The medical assistant asks the patient to disrobe and gown for the visit.

> The medical assistant informs the patient of the approximate wait time for the physician based on the current schedule.

Visit Preparation

> The nurse prepares for the visit by reviewing the last visit note and any tests that were ordered at the last visit and determining clinical intervention that may be needed. This preparation occurs from 3:00 p.m. to 5:00 p.m. the day prior to the visit. For same-day appointments, this preparation occurs at least one hour prior to the patient's scheduled appointment.

> The nurse obtains test results and makes them available to the physician prior to the patient visit.

(Continued on next page)

> ➤ The nurse reviews the patient's outstanding medical issues and any tests that are due; the nurse also reviews the disease registry and other documentation to determine next steps for the patient at least one hour prior to the scheduled visit.
>
> ➤ The nurse anticipates the needs of the physician and patient for the upcoming visit and prepares all forms or potential waivers and referrals that may be needed.
>
> ➤ The nurse prepares the exam room to include laying out supplies needed for the exam.
>
> ➤ The nurse makes sure that the exam room is fully stocked by evaluating the visual cues that have been placed in the drawers and wall pockets and restocks if needed.
>
> ➤ The nurse prepares the patient for the exam. This includes following the established protocols for each patient type and diagnosis, for example, diabetic patients have their shoes and socks removed (and so forth).

STREAMLINED WORK PROCESSES

A number of other books fully describe the patient flow process and streamlined work processes in depth.[4] In this section, we provide an overview of patient-focused work processes to help you identify opportunities to reduce waste and streamline work in your medical practice to benefit physicians, staff, and patients.

Patient-Focused Front Office

➤ Huddle at the beginning of each morning session and again at the beginning of each afternoon session

---

[4] See Woodcock, Elizabeth W. 2009. *Mastering Patient Flow: Using Lean Thinking to Improve Your Practice Operations, 3rd Edition.* Englewood, Colo.: Medical Group Management Association.

> Streamline and ensure friendly retrieval of patients for place-ment in exam rooms (consider the use of paging devices for patients, immediate rooming of the patient, or patient self-rooming)[5]

> Eliminate check-in and/or check-out stations and perform this work in the exam room

> Conduct previsit financial clearance: insurance and eligibility verification, authorizations, time-of-service payment obliga-tions

Patient-Focused Telephones

> Offer multiple access avenues — telephone, Web portal, secure online messaging, virtual visits

> Ensure easy patient access; one-stop service

> Be a financial and personal advocate for the patient

> Respond to patient calls in real time, minimizing messages

> Minimize telephone contact with the patient (offer online scheduling, test-results reporting, and online answers to pa-tient inquiries so patients can communicate with your office at times most convenient for them rather than limit this to office hours when telephones are staffed);

> Anticipate patient needs and provide them with information, for example, when and how they will get their test results and five common questions and answers pertinent to the diagnosis or procedure performed, thereby reducing the need for pa-tients to "go fish" for this information

Patient-Focused Clinical Support

> Prepare for the visit by identifying the reason for visit, out-standing lab/test results; plan outstanding or next step inter-ventions per disease and care registries

---

[5] Patient self-rooming has been introduced at the Park Nicollet Clinic. See "Park Nicollet Health Services Case Studies." In: Black, John, with David Miller. 2008. *The Toyota Way to Healthcare Excellence: Increase Efficiency and Improve Quality with Lean.* Chicago: Health Administration Press.

- Prepare the exam room by stocking it in a precise, predetermined fashion and laying out needed supplies and materials
- Use a standard greeting with patients
- Conduct standard vital signs, medication review, and chief complaint review with the patient
- Prepare the patient by gowning and draping for the physician and explaining next visit steps
- Participate in the visit and populate chart and registry, obtain patient history, and present the patient to the physician[6]
- Discharge the patient from the exam room by providing him or her with a summary of the visit and treatment plan and providing education consistent with the patient's condition

Work Delegation

Delegate to the flow nurse

- Support the visit with concurrent steps (as opposed to sequential steps) in the exam room with the physician
- Provide the patient with a take-home tool
- Assign the patient a health coach or care manager, or identify another method to follow-up with the patient
- Send online message reminders to the patient

Delegate to the phone nurse

- Manage inbound calls in real time
- Manage patient clinical logs to identify outstanding tests and ensure review and reporting of results to the patient
- Manage the Web portal related to secure messages initiated by the patient to the practice

---

[6] Anderson, Peter, and Marc D. Halley. 2008 "A new approach to making your doctor–nurse team more productive." *Fam Pract Manag.* 15(17):35–40. Also see www.familyteamcare.org.

Delegate to the patient

- Develop online patient access via Web portal, with the patient conducting scheduling, registration changes, secure messaging, test results, prescription renewal, and education online

- Provide the ability for patients to update registration information online prior to the visit

- Use a kiosk to permit patients to conduct self check-in for the visit

- Permit patients to travel unescorted to an assigned exam room

SUMMARY

In this chapter, we described lean management systems and lean principles used to create standard work. We also discussed redesigned work processes for staff in the medical practice. The examples in this chapter are just a few of the many work processes that can be selected for redesign and lean principles. The goal is to create intentional discipline in the work, review each process and eliminate waste and non–value-added steps, thereby improving the patient experience and staff efficiency and effectiveness. The care team is then deployed to work with streamlined processes to improve value to patients.

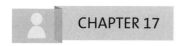

CHAPTER 17

Creating Purposeful Work

...the highest level of individual development and the greatest happiness are derived from serving ends beyond the self — ends that employees value, that enable them to feel they are "making a difference," and consequently that bring increased meaning to their lives through work.

—Leading with Purpose: The New Corporate Realities

By working in a medical practice, you have a distinct advantage. The purpose of your work in healthcare is truly existential. You are providing a service to others, and each and every day you make a difference in people's lives.

In this chapter, we discuss:

> ➤ The importance of purposeful work
>
> ➤ Connecting staff to purpose

WHAT IS OUR PURPOSE?

The purpose of your medical practice is to make a difference in people's lives by helping them maintain or improve their health and wellness. You do meaningful work each and every day. This purpose stimulates employee commitment and creativity. Unfortunately, it is easy to forget our purpose. The day-to-day operational demands of a medical practice often take hold and the following sometimes occurs: when that last patient of the day is checked in, we often do not really see the patient at all; the patient is simply a diagnosis or number 126 of the day. If physicians and staff forget their purpose, you risk losing not only the core competence of your medical practice, but also the meaningfulness of the important work these people play as a member of the care team. The care team loses its enthusiasm and motivation. The work simply becomes a job, not a true profession.

> You do meaningful work each and every day. This purpose stimulates employee commitment and creativity.

CONNECTING STAFF TO PURPOSE

It is important to work to connect the staff to the clinical care and service provided to your patients. This requires attention to job design to emotionally connect the staff to their work; "… when health care workers' jobs are structured so they can treat patients holistically, rather than performing disconnected individual tasks, it enables them to care and be more fully present in their work."[1] It also requires making a specific effort to identify the value-added work that the staff member carries out in service to the patient.

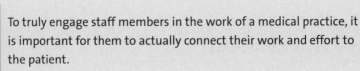

> To truly engage staff members in the work of a medical practice, it is important for them to actually connect their work and effort to the patient.

[1] Burud, Sandra, and Marie Tumolo. 2004. *Leveraging the New Human Capital: Adaptive Strategies, Results Achieved, and Stories of Transformation.* Palo Alto, Calif.: Davies-Black Publishing; p. 31.

When I visit medical practices throughout the country, I have the opportunity to meet with many talented and engaged front office and back office staff. The vast majority of these staff seem happy to share their current work processes, successes, and challenges.

When I ask them to describe what they do, however, I often hear the following:

> ➤ "I collect co-pays."
>
> ➤ "I room the patient."
>
> ➤ "I pull charts."
>
> ➤ "I submit claims."
>
> ➤ "I'm a rad tech."

To truly engage staff members in the work of a medical practice, it is important for them to actually connect their work and effort to the patient. In Exhibit 17.1, look at the different responses from staff in medical practices that have successfully made this connection.

You go to work every day and face significant challenges in a medical practice. Patients are often not at their best — they are ill and frightened and are at times short-tempered and rude. Physicians, too, are often stressed to the max, as they work with a mass of billing paperwork and regulatory requirements that rival that of any other organization. Yet amid this chaos, physicians are required to diagnose and treat illnesses with far-reaching implications — in many instances, it truly is a matter of life or death or quality of that life. Yet most of the board meetings I attend and the physician meetings that I am invited to relate to the business of medicine, not clinical issues. I think we need more discussion of purpose — how you helped Johnny go to school for the first time, how Mrs. Smith was able to celebrate her anniversary, how Mr. Johnson got to walk his daughter down the aisle.

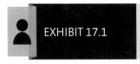 **EXHIBIT 17.1**   Staff Connected to Purposeful Work

Work	Purposeful Work
I collect co-pays.	I welcome patients to the practice and put them at ease. I make sure that patients know how to communicate with the practice, that they understand their insurance plan and know what they need to pay at their visit so they are not surprised.
I room the patient.	I prepare for the patient visit by making sure the exam room and the patient are ready for the physician. I take vital signs and I obtain the latest information regarding the medications and the reason for the visit. I listen to the patient and anticipate his or her needs.
I pull charts.	I make sure patient records are up-to-date and provide the physician, referring physician, and the patient with important healthcare information.
I submit claims.	I am the liaison between the patient and the payer and essentially serve as the patient's financial advocate. I help patients understand what their insurance will and will not pay and serve as a resource to the patients.
I'm a rad tech.	I integrate with the patient visit. When the physician orders an x-ray, I go to the exam room and escort the patient to the x-ray room. I make sure the results are immediately available so that the physician can complete the exam.

The knowledge workers in your medical practices are dual-focus workers.[2] These are individuals who care about the work and, in addition, care about their home life. Work–life balance has taken on a new meaning for today's workers and for today's physicians. The ideal worker is a "multidimensional individual who is effective in dual-focus mode (managing work and personal life simultaneously), can deliver results collaboratively, can innovate and challenge, works well in diverse employment arrangements, and possesses meta-competencies that leverage technical skills: a whole person who can bring heart, mind, and hands to work."[3]

> The knowledge workers in our medical practices are dual-focus workers.

SUMMARY

The purpose of this chapter is simply to remind the reader of our purpose and the importance of connecting your care team members to that purpose. In the midst of chaos, this connection to purpose helps staff make the right decisions for patients and it also reminds them why they chose to work in healthcare in the first place. I certainly can't think of many other professions that bring the rewards you get each and every day as you make a difference in people's lives.

[2] Burud, Sandra, and Marie Tumolo. 2004. *Leveraging the New Human Capital: Adaptive Strategies, Results Achieved, and Stories of Transformation.* Palo Alto, Calif.: Davies-Black Publishing, p. 35.

[3] Ibid; p. 58.

PART 6

Staff Recruitment, Recognition, and Retention

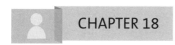

CHAPTER 18

Grow, Hire, Share, or Outsource

But knowledge workers own the means of production. It is the knowledge between their ears. And it is a totally portable and enormous capital asset.

—Peter F. Drucker

The staff in your medical practice are both knowledge and service workers.[1] The intellectual capital required to work in a medical practice resides within the minds of employees. Policy and procedure manuals do not detail how to build an on-call schedule, how to perform nurse triage, or how to determine and collect a patient's deductible. The core competencies of your medical practice are the unique assets of your physicians, nonphysician providers, and staff.

In this chapter, we discuss the opportunities and implications of:

➤ Growing staff

➤ Hiring staff

➤ Sharing staff

➤ Outsourcing work

---

[1] For the combination of knowledge and service workers for today's organizations, see Burud, Sandra, and Marie Tumolo. 2004. *Leveraging the New Human Capital: Adaptive Strategies, Results Achieved, and Stories of Transformation.* Palo Alto, Calif.: Davies-Black Publishing.

GROWING STAFF

One of the primary considerations when there is a staff vacancy is whether to promote from within or to hire from outside the medical practice.

In a number of medical practices, a conscious decision is made to prepare for succession planning and to identify staff for a progressive track within the practice. In this fashion, staff are provided with educational opportunities (growing their expertise) so that they can take on additional breadth and scope of responsibility. The advantages of this approach are many — the staff member's strengths and weaknesses are already apparent to the practice and the staff member has had the opportunity to assimilate the culture of the medical practice.

For succession planning to work, follow these steps:

1. Identify potential stars in the practice.

2. Develop a professional growth plan for these staff that involves additional education and training.

3. Delegate additional responsibilities to these staff, and provide the tools for them to succeed.

4. Work with them one-on-one to improve their decision-making and cognitive skill sets.

5. Consider assigning these staff an intern role to allow them to devote more time to these added responsibilities.

6. Develop a formal mentoring program to target high performers and actively manage their trajectory through the organization.

This approach, which involves growing or educating the staff for additional responsibilities, typically also includes educational programs and support for the staff. For example, tuition reimbursement can be offered for relevant classes or the medical practice can share in the educational costs, with requirements related to earned grade-point average and tenure with the practice. Some medical practices establish scholarship funds for which staff can apply, with criteria for awards related to years with the practice and type of education to be received.

> When a medical practice has a staff vacancy, it is an opportune time to revisit the staffing model. It may be that a new staff member is not needed if a change is made to the existing staffing deployment model.

HIRING STAFF

When you have a staff vacancy in your medical practice, it is an opportune time to revisit your staffing model. It may be that a new staff member is not needed if a change is made to your existing staffing deployment model. Prior to updating the job description and posting the job vacancy, ask and answer the following questions:

➤ What functions and tasks have been delegated to this staff member?

➤ Is there a specific licensure that is needed to perform this work?

➤ Do we need to recruit for this position or is there a different staffing deployment model that we can use in our medical practice to accomplish this work?

➤ As part of this recruitment, can we combine roles and responsibilities in new and different ways, thereby elevating or growing a staff member to this role?

➤ Does the work need to be conducted in the way we have always done it, or is there a new or more innovative way to complete the work that may change our staffing needs?

➤ Is there a better way to accomplish the work responsibilities, such as outsourcing or sharing this role with another practice or another suite?

If the decision is made to hire a new staff member, this is the time to extend and strengthen your care team.

> New employees need to possess the intellectual capital to do the work, as well as the relational and social capital to work in a care team providing service to patients.

Focus on selective recruiting — identifying individuals with skill, talent, and a cultural and value fit with the medical practice. It is important to also hire people who take responsibility for their work and contribute to the organization.[2] New employees need to possess the intellectual capital to do the work, as well as the relational and social capital to work in a care team providing service to patients. Some experts indicate you should emphasize skills and knowledge when you recruit; others indicate you should emphasize culture and teamwork. Ideally, you want both and you want individuals who are innovative, creative, and entrepreneurial and who can think on their feet. Contrast a blank canvas with a paint-by-numbers kit. In medical practices, we need the blank canvas.[3]

Where to Look?

Several approaches should be used concurrently to identify a new staff member for the practice. These include:

- ➤ Leading Internet job sites
- ➤ Medical practice Website and social networking sites

---

[2] See Burud, Sandra, and Marie Tumolo. 2004. *Leveraging the New Human Capital: Adaptive Strategies, Results Achieved, and Stories of Transformation.* Palo Alto, Calif.: Davies-Black Publishing; p. 136, for a discussion of concrete examples of selective recruitment and intensive retention.

[3] The notion of blank canvas and paint-by-numbers was described by Jim Collins, author of *Good to Great* and *Built to Last.* Also, "In Times Like These You Get a Chance to Show Your Strength," Interview with Jim Collins by Bo Bulingham, *Inc. Magazine,* April 2009, p. 81.

- Journal and newspaper advertisements
- Technical schools
- Community colleges and universities
- Job fairs
- Health fairs
- Temporary staff agency (with temporary to full-time staffing)

Many physicians and practice executives report that their best source of new talent is by word of mouth. They communicate job openings to their current staff and their hospital partner. Some medical practices pay the current staff a bonus as a referral fee for a new staff hire with staff using their social networks such as Facebook and LinkedIn to recruit candidates. The approach taken by a medical practice varies based on the local job market and the avenues available for communication and distribution of job vacancy information.

Once applications are received, conduct a formal review of the applications using a standardized review process. Then decide whether an initial screening by social media, telephone, or video interview will be conducted or whether you wish to schedule a face-to-face interview with each qualified applicant.

Interview Questions

Develop standard interview questions and pose the questions to each interviewee. At least three areas of questions should be included:

- Specific knowledge and skills
- Judgment and decision-making abilities
- Behavioral skills

Focus on selective recruiting — identifying individuals with skill, talent, and a cultural and value fit with the medical practice.

Open-ended questions elicit more dialogue with the applicant and provide insights into the applicant's teamwork, attitude, and interpersonal style. Examples of open-ended interview questions are provided in Exhibit 18.1.

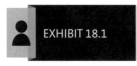

EXHIBIT 18.1   Open-Ended Interview Questions

> ➤ What is it about this job that appeals to you?
> ➤ What skills do you bring that are unique?
> ➤ How would your team members describe your role and contributions?
> ➤ What type of work gives you the most joy?

Behavioral questions permit the applicant to demonstrate or explain specific actions and behaviors he or she would initiate in particular situations. Examples of behavioral interview questions for a medical assistant applicant are provided in Exhibit 18.2.

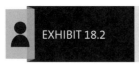

EXHIBIT 18.2   Behavioral Interview Questions

> ➤ Here is a blood pressure cuff. Let's role-play. Pretend I am a patient and please take my blood pressure.
> ➤ The patient is confused regarding the medications she is taking. What action would you take to make sure you have the most up-to-date medication list?
> ➤ Please walk me through the steps you use to prepare for the patient visit.

The Interview

Candidates should undergo interviews with the direct supervisor of the position, as well as a small group of staff. By having a team involved in the interview process, the medical practice reinforces the importance of collaboration and teamwork — team matters. If the staff member is to work directly with a physician, that physician should also be involved in the interview process, either at the first interview opportunity or when the list of candidates has been reduced to two or three.

Prior to Start Date

Once a candidate has been selected, it is important to start the orientation of the staff member before the first day of work. Invite him or her to lunch with a small group of staff and/or share materials regarding the medical practice prior to the first day of work to give the candidate a head start on the job. For example, send the candidate your policy and procedure manual, list of physicians, list of staff, and other important basic material to orient the candidate to the medical practice.

New Staff Orientation

Plan the on-boarding process of new staff. Develop a formal orientation process involving a checklist to ensure that each new staff member receives a complete orientation to the practice and to his or her particular job responsibilities. (Note that the checklist is a form of standard work, consistent with our discussion in Chapter 16, Work Process Redesign.)

Assign a teammate to the new staff member so that he or she has someone to approach with day-to-day questions. The teammate selected for this role should be a high performer in your medical practice. He or she can be tasked with orienting the new staff member to the practice, describing its history and its culture. In addition, it is important to develop a formal process to oversee the work of new staff, until their competency levels are assessed. For example, a new nurse should be assessed on all nursing functions. Similarly, a new patient scheduler or biller should be evaluated to ensure competency on the practice management system prior to permitting him or her to perform independent work.

SHARING STAFF

A number of positions in a medical practice can be shared with another medical practice or with another healthcare organization. Some examples are provided in the following sections.

Practice Executive

It is not uncommon for medical practices to share a practice executive, either as an employee or an independent consultant to the practice. In this fashion, a high-level executive with breadth and scope of expertise can provide broad management support to the practice, interacting with the office manager, supervisor, or lead on a daily or weekly basis. For example, one practice administrator can be shared among five solo or two-physician practices. As another example, a regional practice manager can be assigned to oversee four or six medical practices. In this fashion, even small medical practices are able to secure the services of a high-level executive or manager in a fiscally appropriate fashion. In addition, the executive is more likely to be fulfilled by having a breadth and scope of responsibility consistent with his or her expertise.

Information Technology Manager

An information technology (IT) manager is another position that is commonly shared among medical practices. This permits a medical practice to have the expertise in-house required for its practice management software, its internal computer network, its Website, and/or its electronic health records. This can take the form of a single manager or a few IT support staff, or it can be expanded to include an entire IT team, each member having specific knowledge and skill for one or more hardware and software applications of the medical practice. By sharing this resource, each medical practice can take advantage of the sophisticated expertise of an IT manager (or team), while appropriately managing its costs for the work.

Billing Manager

Today's physician billing process is complex, and it is prudent to have sophisticated billing expertise at the helm. This can be accomplished by sharing a billing manager with another practice, thereby permitting each practice to have the insights and expertise of a sophisticated billing manager without bearing the full cost of this position. A knowledgeable and experienced billing manager can also reduce the business risk in a medical practice, given the heightened knowledge of national, state, and payer rules and regulations required for today's revenue cycle, and avoid the "potholes" in the road to getting paid.[4]

Ancillary Staff

Many medical practices want the convenience of offering ancillary services onsite, yet do not have the patient volume to make this feasible. Sharing ultrasound technologists, imaging technicians, phlebotomists, and other ancillary staff can be instituted, providing a shared resource for multiple medical practices (provided all legal and regulatory issues are attended to). Similarly, a dietician, a diabetic nurse coordinator, and other specialty roles can be shared with other medical practices.

OUTSOURCING WORK

Outsourcing staff work functions can also extend the staffing model of a medical practice. Examples of outsourcing opportunities are provided in the following sections.

---

[4] See Walker Keegan, Deborah L.; Elizabeth W. Woodcock; and Sara M. Larch. 2009. *The Physician Billing Process: 12 Potholes to Avoid in the Road to Getting Paid*. Englewood, Colo.: Medical Group Management Association.

Professional Fee Billing and Collection

Vendors can provide the full scope of back-end billing, typically defined as the steps after charge entry. Alternatively, they can perform specific billing functions and tasks. For example:

> ➤ *Patient collections.* Collection agencies are now taking on added roles related to patient account follow-up on outstanding patient balances, up to and including the traditional role of follow-up with patients for delinquent payments.

> ➤ *Insurance account follow-up.* Outstanding accounts receivable can be outsourced to a vendor to follow up with payers. Medical practices typically use such vendors as an adjunct to in-house follow-up efforts.

> ➤ *Payment posting.* Banks and lockbox services are expanding their role in financial support to medical practices. Patient payments, in particular, can be posted by the lockbox service, with an electronic file of payments posted to the practice management system. The staff in the medical practice are thus freed up to devote their time to examining reimbursement levels and conducting account follow-up rather than simply entering payments into the practice management system.

> ➤ *Coding.* Coding vendors provide enhanced coding knowledge specific to each specialty in the medical practice to ensure appropriate procedure coding for rendered services.

Information Technology

Everything from Website management to electronic health records support can be outsourced to a vendor serving as a virtual IT department of the medical practice.

Duplication and Scanning

Vendors are available to duplicate and scan medical records, thereby permitting full-time staff to be devoted to other obligations that typically require more sophisticated expertise.

Accounting

Many medical practices outsource their accounting and taxation duties to a knowledgeable vendor. In this fashion, the on-site practice executive is freed up for other tasks.

Payroll

Other medical practices partner with a human resources outsourcing firm or administrative services organization to manage payroll and to pay the appropriate payroll taxes and benefit costs, thereby freeing up financial staff in the medical practice to focus on other areas, such as revenue cycle management.

These are just a few examples of the many work functions that can be considered for outsourcing.

SUMMARY

In this chapter, we discussed key issues associated with growing and developing current staff for additional responsibilities, hiring staff to the care team, sharing staff with other organizations or parts of the organization, and outsourcing work to a vendor partner. We discussed the importance of evaluating your current staffing deployment model to determine if changes to the model are warranted. Through this process, the medical practice is continually evaluating its staffing model to innovate and ensure alignment.

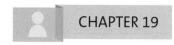

CHAPTER 19

Talent Management: Nurse Betty Behaving Badly

Management is about human beings. Its task is to make people capable of joint performance, to make their strengths effective and their weaknesses irrelevant.

—The Definitive Drucker

Everyone is good, and no one is too good.

—Tom H. Stearns, FACMPE
Vice President, Medical Practice Services
State Volunteer Mutual Insurance Company

We all seem to have them at one time or another — a staff member who is simply not a good fit for the team. In many cases, we walk on eggshells around these staff and try to avoid them in the interest of office harmony. This approach often backfires as we come to realize that the staff member who behaves badly or acts out is like a "cancer" in the practice, disrupting the best efforts of others and actually holding back team talent and progress.

What keeps us up at night is not the latest, greatest changes to the Stark Law or the latest, greatest changes to physician billing or patient scheduling, but the human resources challenges that weigh most heavily on our minds. At times we make the unfortunate mistake of being so afraid to be short-staffed that we retain problem employees who cannot multitask, don't jump in to offer to help others, and are not team players. Yet, they are loyal or they are long-term, so we tolerate their aberrant behavior. The real question we should be asking about these staff is, are they adding value to the practice?

In this chapter, we discuss:

➤ Performance expectations

➤ The talent management process

➤ Rewarding positive performance with positive rewards

➤ Staff education plans

> The real question we should be asking about these staff is, are they adding value to the practice?

PERFORMANCE EXPECTATIONS

It is important for each medical practice to articulate the performance expected of its staff and to expect high levels of talent and contribution. For example, in addition to specific skills and knowledge required for a position, most of us want staff to demonstrate the following:

➤ *Team orientation.* A staff member who is an integral, active part of the care team

➤ *Continuous improvement.* A staff member who helps redesign processes to eliminate waste

➤ *Decision-making and judgment.* A staff member who is able to think on his or her feet and make good decisions

➤ *Self-management.* A staff member who does not require strict oversight and who demonstrates awareness of self and understanding of his or her strengths and areas in need of improvement

➤ *Customer service.* A staff member who is able to put patients at ease and provide quality service

➤ *Communication.* A staff member who demonstrates an effective interpersonal communication style

Develop a formal list of the behaviors and talents that you expect your staff to demonstrate. If you do not articulate what is expected, you cannot hold staff accountable to the expectations and likely will not get the behaviors and talents you want. The key to talent management is holding individuals accountable for performance and results.

THE TALENT MANAGEMENT PROCESS

There are full texts devoted to staff performance management. In this book, we touch on some key elements to consider when evaluating talent in a medical practice and draw attention to some components that are often overlooked.

Define the formal process you will use to conduct staff performance review. This process should outline the who, what, when, and how a staff member is evaluated in the medical practice and the performance expectations of the staff. There are a number of different performance management processes used in medical practices, including:

➤ *Top-down and bottom-up.* Some medical practices ask the staff to review their job descriptions and note their areas of strengths, weaknesses, and accomplishments. The supervisor then meets with the staff to review these self-reported evaluations and provides input. Together, a formal evaluation is prepared.

➤ *Physician–administrator.* Some medical practices ask the physicians for input, with the supervisor combining this information with his or her own to develop a formal evaluation that is reviewed with the staff member.

➤ *360-degree assessments.* Some medical practices have expanded to 360-degree assessment instruments (or a more limited approach). In these practices, colleagues, patients, physicians, and/or staff in other units are asked to provide input regarding the performance of staff in the medical practice. The supervisor and staff member review this feedback, and together prepare a formal evaluation.

> The key to talent management is holding individuals accountable for performance and results.

Regardless of the method that is employed, it is important that the talent management process include:

- Performance and talent expectations of the staff member
- Assessment of the staff member's performance and talent in relation to the expectations
- Analysis of strengths
- Analysis of weaknesses or areas that need improvement
- Future goals and expectations
- Staff education and development plan
- Feedback from the staff on what they feel they need in order to do their best work

This last point — feedback from the staff on what they need from management — is often overlooked by medical practices. The role of management is to provide the tools and support for staff to perform their very best work. The manager's role is to ensure that the staff have the tools and support needed for them to exercise their strengths and ensure that the work is matched to those strengths.

If the medical practice embraces this management role, then either 360-degree assessment instruments or career satisfaction assessments should be used to gauge the impact of the work environment on staff. These can be administered as part of the talent review process or at established intervals in a medical practice. An example of a career satisfaction instrument is provided in Exhibit 19.1.

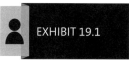

EXHIBIT 19.1   Career Satisfaction Instrument

Area	Not Satisfied	Satisfied	More Than Satisfied
Assigned work and tasks			
Professional career goals			
Financial rewards			
Nonfinancial rewards			
Communication			
Access to management			
Relationship with supervisor			
Team member interaction			
Work resources and tools			
Continuous learning opportunity			
Balance of work/life			
Care team effectiveness			

What additional tools, resources, and/or support would improve your ability to provide your best work and talent to the care team?

The manager's role is to ensure that the staff have the tools and support needed for them to exercise their strengths.

Assessing the talent of staff in your medical practice not only requires up-to-date job descriptions that outline expected work functions and tasks, but also the outcomes expected of the staff. Use the expected staff workload ranges that we shared in Chapter 5, The Staff Workload Evaluation Process, and in the chapters on staffing each key component of the medical practice as specific expectations regarding work quantity. Coupled with expectations regarding work quality, these can form the basis of performance expectations for the care team.

A typical rating schedule for staff performance includes four levels: unsatisfactory or significantly below standards, improvement needed, satisfactory, and more than satisfactory. The specific functions and behaviors required for each of these ratings should be pre-established. Examples of expectations required to receive More Than Satisfactory evaluations are provided in Exhibits 19.2 and 19.3. In Exhibit 19.2, the performance expectations for Teamwork and Initiative are detailed. Exhibit 19.3 details the performance expectations for Telephone Management.

Adopt a similar approach to define in advance the specific performance expectations required of your staff. There should be no surprises at the time of the performance review. That is, the staff member should have been provided with the performance expectations in advance and, additionally, the staff member should have received continuous feedback regarding his or her performance throughout the year, not only at year-end.

By assessing staff talent, work quantity, and work quality, we can directly see the staff member's contribution to the care team, as depicted in Exhibit 19.4.

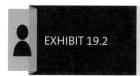

EXHIBIT 19.2

Teamwork and Initiative:
Performance Expectation to Receive
More Than Satisfactory

➤ **Supports medical practice goals and values**

Exemplifies medical practice goals and values through
words and actions

➤ **Exhibits objectivity and openness to others' viewpoints**

Welcomes the opinions and views of others; always
maintains a high degree of objectivity

➤ **Exhibits tact and consideration**

Consistently tactful and considerate in relations with others

➤ **Contributes to building a positive team spirit**

A leader in building a strong team spirit and identity

➤ **Steps in to help teammates when needed**

Demonstrates initiative and volunteers immediately
when sees that help is needed

➤ **Respects others' work time**

Consistently aware of others' workloads and takes special
care not to disrupt

➤ **Makes decisions that reflect a patient-focused care team**

Consistently makes decisions of high quality and exercises
judgment in support of the patient

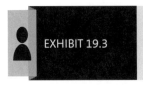

EXHIBIT 19.3

Telephone Management:
Performance Expectation to Receive
More Than Satisfactory

> ➤ **Answers telephone within three rings**
>
> Consistently treats callers as a priority and demonstrates a high work volume; is extremely efficient and effective at handling inbound telephone calls
>
> ➤ **Uses standard greeting**
>
> Consistently uses standard greeting, assists others to do so, and makes certain that the greeting is genuine to the patient
>
> ➤ **Demonstrates telephone courtesy**
>
> Is exceptionally caring, warm, and efficient in telephone manner
>
> ➤ **Demonstrates empathy and concern in call management**
>
> Demonstrates empathy, yet is able to respond to the caller in an efficient fashion; extremely efficient in managing large call volume; accurately responds to patient inquiries within work scope
>
> ➤ **Takes accurate messages**
>
> Records exceptionally legible, accurate, and complete messages; consistently gets information needed to facilitate call resolution
>
> ➤ **Keeps the service promise and practices service recovery**
>
> Consistently gets back to patients the same day to advise them of status and goes the extra mile to recover from service deficits caused by the practice
>
> ➤ **Exercises judgment in difficult situations**
>
> Demonstrates excellent judgment and initiative in managing difficult patients and sensitive situations

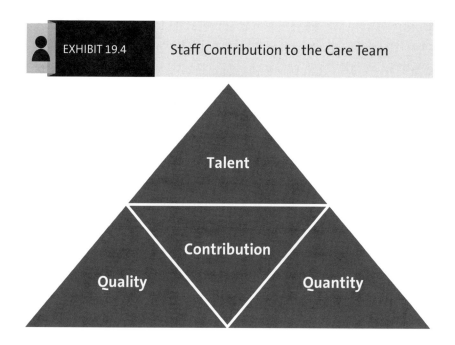

EXHIBIT 19.4   Staff Contribution to the Care Team

REWARDING POSITIVE PERFORMANCE WITH POSITIVE REWARDS

It is also important to recognize that as we assess the talent and contribution of staff, we often make the mistake of inappropriate linkages between performance and consequences. We "reward A, while hoping for B."[1] It is important to link the right performance with the right consequences. For example, poor performance should be met with negative consequences, and good performance should be met with positive consequences.[2]

---

[1] Kerr, Steven. 1975. "On the folly of rewarding A, while hoping for B." *Acad Manage J.* 18(4):769–783.

[2] The author wishes to acknowledge Chris Hipple, University Physicians Inc., University of Maryland School of Medicine for this distinction and her work in this area.

Unfortunately, we often see an inappropriate linkage between performance and consequences. Consider the following examples:

➤ *Nurse Betty Behaving Badly.* Nurse Betty is a difficult employee. When a project is due, the manager decides to delegate it to Nurse Superstar rather than Nurse Betty. It is just too difficult to work with Nurse Betty, so she is not asked to take on these additional duties, which demand long hours and increased work levels.

– In this example, Betty's poor performance receives a positive consequence. She is not asked to take on added roles and responsibilities, nor is she asked to work extended hours.

➤ *Supervisor Sally is Terrific.* There is a new position available for which Sally qualifies, and it would mean a promotion for her. Rather than recommend her for this new position, however, the manager decides to hire from outside the practice.

– In this example, Sally is viewed as too valuable to promote to the next level. This is an example of good talent receiving negative consequences.

Evaluate your day-to-day management style to ensure that performance and consequence are consistent. Be sure that an unintended mismatch is not routine; positive behavior should receive positive rewards and negative behavior should receive negative consequences.

Experts strongly suggest that companies pay specific attention to their high performers — known as HiPos.[3] High performers are increasingly frustrated, as they often take on more than their fair share of work in a medical practice and they may see limited advancement opportunity. To engage HiPos, some companies assign difficult problems to the high performers for them to solve, others ask their best staff to attend strategy meetings and take an active role in setting strategic direction. These organizations are combining such HiPo

---

[3] Schumpeter. 2002. "Overstretched. Many people who keep their jobs are working too hard. What can companies do about it?" *The Economist.* Business Section, May 22, 2010, p. 72.

schemes with lay-offs and terminations of low-performing staff, recognizing that "most workers are surprisingly keen on rewarding superstars and on dumping freeloaders."[4] An inability to correctly link performance with appropriate consequences often leads to low staff morale for the best and the brightest staff in the medical practice.

STAFF EDUCATION PLANS

"The best learning comes from a combination of experience, hands-on training, and mentoring, with explicit feedback loops."[5]

A formal staff education plan for the medical practice is needed. Particularly if the local job market does not have a wealth of medical practice operations talent, a formal internal education program will develop staff and maintain knowledge currency. Take the following steps when developing a staff education plan:

1. Create a formal training program for each functional area.

2. Identify national and local resources for the particular functional area to assist with education and ongoing updates.

3. Identify seminars, tools, Webinars, audioconferences, online education, and reading material and plan for staff to participate. Ask staff to bring back key information to share with the team.

4. Hold regular staff meetings and assign staff to become experts in particular areas, such as advanced access scheduling, collections at the point of care, methods to manage patients with multiple chronic conditions, best practices in patient flow, and other similar important work. Expect staff to expand current knowledge of the medical practice and bring suggestions to change work processes to staff meetings.

---

[4] Ibid.
[5] Edersheim, Elizabeth Haas. 2007. *The Definitive Drucker*. New York: McGraw-Hill; p. 180.

5. Conduct formal competency assessments of staff and use these to identify additional educational needs for the care team.

6. Hold dedicated training days (or portions of the day) to discuss focused topics. Make sure adult learning is supported; actively engage the staff in the education, rather than simply use a didactic approach.

DEVELOPING PROFESSIONAL SKILLS AND BEHAVIORS IN SUPPORT STAFF

Professional performance underlies the ability of a medical practice to operate efficiently and effectively. Professional behaviors result from institutionalizing the values of the organization, developing clear performance expectations, providing education and development opportunities, and providing ongoing assessment of behavior in the context of organizational expectations. A framework and model for professional skills development are provided in Exhibits 19.5 and 19.6.

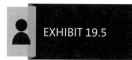

EXHIBIT 19.5   Framework for Professional Skills Development

I. **Institutionalize Expected Behaviors**

    a. Define the vision and philosophy

    b. Define values and expectations of the medical practice

    c. Create a quality and service orientation

    d. Become who we are, not what we want to be like

II. **Build Responsibility at All Levels**

    a. Define performance expectations

    b. Determine education and development needs

    c. Build management skills to support the changing expectations

    d. Obtain staff input and expect involvement

    e. Delegate decisions to others

    f. Create management identity as a team

III. **Evaluate and Continually Assess Progress**

    a. Evaluate behavior based on performance expectations

    b. Evaluate skills based on performance expectations

    c. Institutionalize involvement by aligning appropriate reward structures

    d. Test whether behavior has been institutionalized

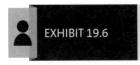

EXHIBIT 19.6 Model for Professional Skills Development

I. Create an Event to Draw Attention to Changing Expectations

    a. Meeting of managers/supervisors to define goals, changing philosophy, and expectations

    b. Meeting of staff to define goals, philosophy, and expectations

    c. Reason for event — for example, changing healthcare delivery system and healthcare reform

    d. Sample event topics:

        i. Where the medical practice has been and where it is going

        ii. Accomplishments to date

        iii. Invaluable role of staff in accomplishments

        iv. Change in philosophy

        v. General staff expectations — professional, care team; patient-centered work; expectations for problem-solving; expectations for following through with promises to colleagues and patients

        vi. Obtain staff input to barriers in their jobs and ideas for solutions

Note: You will be creating expectations for change. You need to be certain to follow through with actions.

II. Initial Focus on Managers/Supervisors

    a. Managers/supervisors to serve as role models for the changing philosophy and expectations

        i. Schedule retreat away from the medical practice

        ii. Define retreat expectations

(Continued on next page)

      iii. Identify manager needs

      iv. Define performance expectations

      v. Change the talent management process and rewards

      vi. Schedule education and development sessions

      vii. Work on problems that impact the entire practice

III. Focus on Support Staff

  a. Carry out the same process as with managers/supervisors

  b. Define session expectations

  c. Identify needs

  d. Define performance expectations

  e. Evaluate based on performance expectations and reward appropriate performance

  f. Charge staff with development of problem-solving strategies and process improvement related to their work functions

IV. Assess Outcomes

  a. Help build a record of successes and share examples of change in culture

  b. Continuously assess whether behavior has been institutionalized, for example, ask new staff to describe the medical practice philosophy, examine staff attitudes, examine patient interactions, examine relationships among care team members

      i. Schedule meetings with current and new staff

      ii. Assess joint project efforts

      iii. Conduct patient interaction surveys

      iv. Tune in to daily communications

  c. Continuously assess staff skill levels and identify needs in education and development

The focus for today's staff has changed to look something like Exhibit 19.7.

As we discussed in Chapter 6, Creating a Care Team, the leader's role is more than simply staying out of the way. The medical practice executive should define the desired outcomes, provide support to the staff, and enable them to live up to their potential, eliminating barriers along the way. Sometimes difficult decisions come with that role, but Nurse Betty Behaving Badly is not something that should be tolerated in any organization.

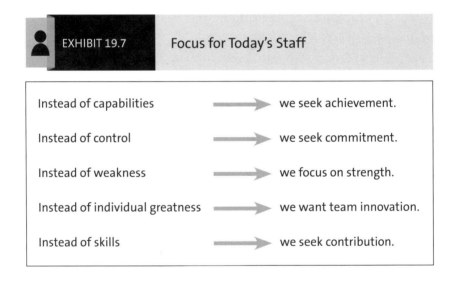

EXHIBIT 19.7   **Focus for Today's Staff**

Instead of capabilities	we seek achievement.
Instead of control	we seek commitment.
Instead of weakness	we focus on strength.
Instead of individual greatness	we want team innovation.
Instead of skills	we seek contribution.

SUMMARY

In this chapter, we discussed the importance of identifying performance expectations and then holding staff members accountable. Talent management is the responsibility of each manager and supervisor in a medical practice. It is not an easy job. It is much easier to overlook Nurse Betty Behaving Badly than to actually address her behavior so that she becomes a contributing member of the care team or is asked to leave the practice. But our failure to address Nurse Betty is a damaging precedent to set for a medical practice and it undermines team success. Expect high levels of contribution, hold staff accountable to that expectation, and help staff become their very best selves.

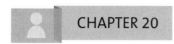

CHAPTER 20

Staff Compensation and Incentive Plans

The role of the medical practice leader is to design the best combination of tangible and intangible rewards that will both recognize employee performance and actively engage employees in implementing change.

—Deborah Walker Keegan, PhD, FACMPE

Human resource experts report that a focus on salary or material inducements to recruit and retain staff misses the mark. In fact, salary is often ranked low on the list of motivating factors reported by staff. Instead, staff are interested in the meaningfulness of the work, trust and relationships among colleagues, ability to balance work and home life, and how they are treated in the workplace — the intangible benefits of working in the medical practice.

In this chapter, we introduce these topics and discuss approaches to staff compensation and incentive plan development, leaving a thorough discussion of these issues to human resource experts and texts (see the Additional Resources section of this book).

In this chapter, we explore:

- ➤ Knowledge workers
- ➤ Components of staff compensation, including base salary and bonus and incentive plans

KNOWLEDGE WORKERS

The staff in a medical practice are knowledge and service workers. They are highly portable — they possess the intellectual capital to do the work and they can walk right across town to another medical practice, taking all of their training and experience with them. Essentially, the staff are free agents; they own the means of their production.[1]

The challenge in knowledge work is to determine how to best measure productivity. Productivity in knowledge work goes beyond the quantity of work to emphasize the quality of that work. The core competency of a medical practice rests with the productivity and quality of its physicians and staff. When staff are paid a flat salary or a flat dollar per hour payment, they are actually being rewarded for time, not productivity, and certainly not for the quality of the work and their contribution to the care team.

> The challenge in knowledge work is to determine how to best measure productivity.

Recognizing this limitation of a flat salary approach to compensation, many medical practices have implemented incentive plans for their staff and/or have worked to include intangible rewards to recognize staff for their talent and contribution.

COMPONENTS OF STAFF COMPENSATION

Staff compensation involves three separate components: salary (or wages), bonus or incentive, and employee benefits. The bonus or incentive component can be further broken down into tangible and intangible rewards. The components of compensation are reported

---

[1] Drucker, Peter F. 1990. *Managing the Nonprofit Organization: Principles and Practices.* New York: Collins Business.

in Exhibit 20.1, and each component is further described in the following sections.

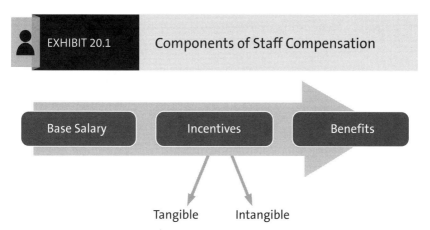

EXHIBIT 20.1   **Components of Staff Compensation**

Base Salary   Incentives   Benefits

Tangible   Intangible

Base Salary

The base salary should be consistent with the skills and knowledge required for the position and for the breadth and scope of the job. It should also be consistent with the local market. Many better-performing medical practices will often pay wage rates that are higher than market rates in order to attract and retain staff, yet they will often also expect more from the staff in terms of engagement and contribution.

Increases to the base salary are made based on a variety of approaches, depending on the medical practice. These include:

> *Market analysis.* A market analysis may periodically be conducted. If such a study indicates that salary levels are below market, a one-time adjustment to the salary for the specific staff involved may be made.

> *Merit increase.* Some medical practices identify a set dollar amount or a set percentage of base salary that is paid as an annual merit increase. Typically, this merit increase becomes a permanent addition to the base salary. So, for example, a medical practice could indicate that it is paying from 1 to

3 percent of base salary as a merit increase. Those who do not meet the performance expectations may receive no merit increase, with progressive payments from 1 to 3 percent of base salary, depending on the annual performance evaluation.

➤ *Cost-of-living adjustment.* Some medical practices attempt to build in a cost-of-living adjustment. A cost-of-living adjustment is not standard in today's medical practices. Declining reimbursement and the financial model on which many medical practices are built make this difficult to sustain over time.

➤ *Range-step advancement.* Some medical practices have identified a salary range and steps within that range. A new staff member with limited work experience may start at the first step in the range, with step increases (and consequently additional salary) earned over time. The step increases may take the place of merit increases and/or they may be additive, depending on the medical practice.

➤ *Level payments.* Some organizations articulate a formula to define a specific level for each employee.[2] Each employee assigned to that level receives the same salary. Thus, for example, the formula may include experience, scope of responsibility, and skill set, with variation producing a 1 to 10 scale of competency. All employees who qualify at level 3 receive the same salary, and so forth.

Bonus and Incentive Plans

In today's medical practices, there is a shift away from permanent increases to the base salary due to the financial model of many medical practices and the uncertainty regarding payer reimbursement. Rather than increase the base salary, many medical practices are moving to bonus or incentive plans for their staff. The incentives consist of tangible rewards and/or intangible rewards. The tangible rewards can be further distinguished into two types: monetary rewards and nonmonetary rewards, as reflected in Exhibit 20.2.

---

[2] Spolsky, Joel. "Why I never let employees negotiate pay raises."*Software, Inc.*, April 2009, pp. 37–38.

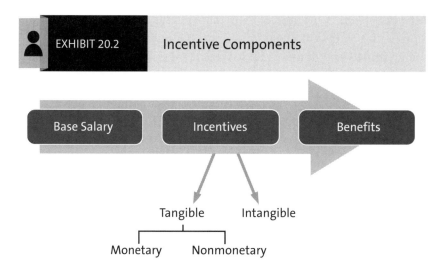

EXHIBIT 20.2   **Incentive Components**

Base Salary   Incentives   Benefits

Tangible   Intangible

Monetary   Nonmonetary

Tangible, Monetary Rewards

Tangible rewards that are monetary are typically detailed in a formal bonus or incentive plan for the medical practice. Incentive plans can be simple, more moderate, or complex, as demonstrated by the following examples.

Simple Plan: An example of a simple plan is for staff to receive a flat dollar level based on hours worked or receive a percentage of base salary each year as a bonus payment. In some medical practices, the bonus comes at holiday time, and the staff are not informed what they did or needed to do in order to earn it. Thus, it becomes an entitlement and an expectation each year. Many medical practices are recognizing that this annual holiday bonus is not effective as an incentive for work. They may continue with a holiday gift, such as a gift card or some dollar figure multiplied by the hours worked. For example, if the multiple is $5.00, a 40-hour-per-week employee receives $200, while a 20-hour-per-week employee receives $100. However, this is viewed as a gift only, not a formal incentive or bonus. For a simple plan to work as an incentive, the specific performance that needs to be met to earn the additional dollars should be articulated in advance and shared with the staff.

Moderate Plan: A number of medical practices have replaced their simple plan with a moderate plan. Specific outcomes and targets are identified and, if met, a bonus or incentive is paid to the staff. Examples of moderate plans include:

> ➤ *Profit sharing approach.* Sharing of annual profitability with the staff based on seniority in the practice, base salary level, or hours worked.

> ➤ *Cost savings approach.* Annual staff costs are budgeted. The cost savings associated with staff turnover, reduction in overtime payments, and other similar staff expenditures are shared with the staff based on seniority, base salary level, or hours worked.

Complex Plan: A complex incentive plan involves multiple targets and goals and may consist of a collection of measures at the individual, team, specialty, or medical practice level.

Here are four examples of complex incentive plans:[3]

Complex Plan A

A specific incentive plan is designed for each type of staff in the medical practice. For example, the telephone staff have one type of incentive plan, the nursing staff have another, the billing staff have a third, and so forth. The work of the staff is evaluated by sampling key functions and tasks, with a portion of the incentive paid for individual performance and a second portion based on group or team performance.

An example of this type of plan for telephone schedulers involves identifying a specific dollar amount to be paid for individual performance and for team performance. For example, telephone staff are eligible to receive both individual and team performance bonuses for a total of $250 per quarter. Each quarter, $125 is available for individual performance and $125 is available for team performance.

---

[3] Adapted with permission from Walker Keegan, Deborah L.; Elizabeth W. Woodcock; and Sara M. Larch. 2009. *The Physician Billing Process: 12 Potholes to Avoid in the Road to Getting Paid.* Englewood, Colo.: Medical Group Management Association.

The individual bonus amount is awarded for the following performance outcomes:

- ➤ "Mystery" calls to telephone operator result in 100 percent compliance with salutation and greeting
- ➤ "Mystery" calls to telephone operator result in 100 percent compliance with patient scheduling policies and procedures
- ➤ A review of 25 sample messages pulled at random results in 100 percent of messages complete and accurate

To receive the $125 that is available for team performance, the performance outcomes include:

- ➤ Percent of inbound telephones calls answered within three rings
- ➤ Call abandonment rate less than 3 percent
- ➤ Patient satisfaction scores related to telephone access at a level of 4 or higher (on a 1 to 5 scale)

As demonstrated in this example, a combination of individual and team incentives is used to provide financial recognition and rewards for telephone management and performance.

Complex Plan B

In this plan, individuals are able to earn up to 10 percent of their gross salary each year based on individual, team, and medical practice goals.

- ➤ Sixty percent of the plan is tied to the individual's performance based on his or her job-specific competencies; the medical practice identifies individual goals at the beginning of the year. Based on the individual's performance, the employee can earn zero to 6 percent of his or her gross salary. The employee must attain a minimum level of individual performance before she or he is eligible for the team or total medical practice incentive.
- ➤ The team (or specialty) incentive is 30 percent of the bonus plan and is tied to team performance. Specific measures are

weighted in importance, such as patient visit volume, patient satisfaction, wait time to appointment, and telephone answering rate. The team incentive criteria are not tied together, so a staff member can be eligible for a portion of the team incentive. For example, if the patient satisfaction target is met and none of the other targets are reached, the staff could still receive a portion of the bonus.

➤ The final goal measures a performance outcome that applies to the entire medical practice. The incentive payment equals 10 percent of the potential incentive. In this example, the incentive is based on overall net collections because the medical practice has to collect enough cash to fund the incentive pool. The practice-wide goal is a stretch goal for the entire group and is not always reached.

Complex Plan C

In this incentive plan, all staff in the medical practice participate, with a variety of measures used to balance the performance and outcomes desired by the medical practice. Point values are listed below for this example; however, these plans can also include various weights and specific targets associated with subcomponents of the performance measure. For example, patient satisfaction survey results can be further distinguished to two or three specific questions on the survey, with each question weighted and a formal target assigned. Below is an example of a balanced set of measures identified for incentive payment:

Performance	*Points*
Patient satisfaction survey results	20
Claim preadjudication errors/edits	20
Time-of-service collections	20
Noncontractual adjustments	10
Net collection rate	15
Accounts receivable >90 days	15
Total points that may be earned	100

A goal is established for each performance area and points are awarded if the medical practice reaches the goals. Dollars per point are determined and communicated to staff each quarter based on the profit level from the previous quarter.

Complex Plan D

In this incentive plan, different practice sites are evaluated and then compared with each other. Each staff member at each site is evaluated with a low, moderate, or high assessment for the following:

- Teamwork
- Customer service
- Financial performance
- Innovation and/or contribution

> In today's medical practices, there is a shift away from permanent increases to the base salary due to the financial model of many medical practices and the uncertainty regarding payer reimbursement.

Incentive Plan Development

Incentive plans can be simple, moderate, or complex. The key is to ensure that the development process for the incentive plan is detailed and thorough, and includes examination of any unintended consequences that might arise.

Be sure to address the following questions as you design an incentive plan for your medical practice:[4]

- What is the objective? What are we trying to accomplish with the incentive plan?

---

[4] Sections of this chapter are adapted with permission from Walker Keegan, Deborah L.; Elizabeth W. Woodcock; and Sara M. Larch. 2009. *The Physician Billing Process: 12 Potholes to Avoid in the Road to Getting Paid*. Englewood, Colo.: Medical Group Management Association.

➤ Do we want to reward individual performance, team performance, or both?

➤ Should the plan reward short-term or long-term goals?

➤ Do we want to provide only tangible rewards or do we need a concerted plan for intangible rewards as well?

➤ Should the incentive plan be constructed with tangible, monetary rewards or tangible, nonmonetary rewards or both?

➤ What specific performance should we measure, monitor, and reward?

➤ Who is eligible to receive the incentive? Should all staff be eligible or only those staff who have met certain criteria, such as years of service or above-average work performance?

➤ What payment method should be used? Should staff receive a flat dollar amount, a percentage of base salary, a share of profitability related to targets and goals, or some other method?

➤ When should the awards be given? Should the rewards be granted monthly, quarterly, or at year-end? Will a delay in rewards permit the staff to connect the reward with their performance?

➤ Should the incentive program be rolled out as a pilot for one year (to ensure it meets its intended goals), or should the plan be put into place with no definable timeline?

➤ How will we finance the incentive plan? What if we fall short of our goals?

➤ What are some unintended consequences that we may see with this incentive plan? How will we respond if they emerge?

➤ Should staff be involved in designing the plan?

➤ How will we communicate the plan to staff?

Regular review of the performance expectations is necessary to keep the plan current. Most medical practices' priorities do change over time, and you want your incentive plans aligned with your medical practice.

By carefully crafting an incentive plan for your medical practice, you can work to avoid unintended consequences.

Unintended Consequences of Incentive Plans

We have witnessed a number of incentive plans that have resulted in unintended consequences. For example, a transcriptionist is awarded additional incentives for work quantity, yet the quality of the work is not incorporated into the incentive determination. As another example, a billing unit is awarded an incentive based on the number of accounts worked, regardless of the quality of action taken on the account. By carefully crafting an incentive plan for your medical practice, you can work to avoid these types of unintended consequences.

Tangible, Nonmonetary Rewards

Tangible rewards that do not involve a monetary payment fall under the category of tangible, nonmonetary rewards. These rewards vary considerably and can range from lunch provided at the practice site, to movie or theatre tickets, to spa memberships, to veterinary benefits, to extra days off work, to a free trip after 10 years of service for two anywhere in the world.

There are four keys to effectively using tangible, nonmonetary rewards:

- Ensure that staff understand what they need to do to earn the reward
- Ensure that the level of reward is consistent with employees' work and effort
- Ensure that the staff value the reward
- Ensure that the administration of the reward is equitable

We have witnessed instances where these types of rewards have backfired:

➤ One medical practice gave each employee a free turkey at Thanksgiving. Employees did not value the free turkey and it came to represent a comedy, with staff equating the level of appreciation for their efforts to that of a turkey.

➤ A medical practice achieved a successful conversion of its practice management system. The administrator placed bags of candy on each employee's desk. This "reward" was viewed as inconsistent with the level of effort and work involved in this project and it backfired.

➤ A practice administrator gave movie tickets to staff to reward them for a job well done. Unfortunately, when the administrator emerged from her office to find the jobs well done, she often missed those staff who had performed admirably at other times during the day when she was not present.

As these examples demonstrate, the use of tangible, nonmonetary rewards should be carefully planned, with attention to the four keys to effectiveness.

Tangible, nonmonetary rewards often can be described as a benefit of working in the medical practice. They are different from the traditional benefits of health insurance, disability, retirement, vacation, and sick leave, and include the following:

➤ Child care services

➤ Flexible work schedules

➤ Notes of appreciation (which I tend to find posted in staff cubicles as sources of pride in their work)

➤ Working remotely

➤ Travel

➤ Health club membership

➤ Spa membership

➤ Aesthetic surgery (one plastic surgery practice offers a free aesthetic procedure to the staff each year, up to $5,000 per person)

➤ Veterinary benefits

➤ After 10 years of service, a two-week vacation for two any place in the world

➤ College tuition support

➤ Masseuse (who comes to the office on Wednesdays)

➤ Dry-cleaning pick-up and delivery

➤ Automobile cleaning and detailing (while you work)

➤ Food (in many medical practices food is abundant)

Intangible Rewards

When we ask why employees love their jobs, we rarely hear them cite their salary. Instead, they cite the intangibles, for example, how well they work with their supervisor or colleagues, their love for patients and the purpose of their work, or the positive environment in which they work. You want to ensure that your best staff elect to stay with you. Studies on employee turnover yield the following top reasons for staff electing to leave their employment:[5]

➤ Lack of growth and development

➤ Insufficient reward and recognition

➤ Did not feel efforts were appreciated

To improve retention of the best and the brightest employees, experts advocate three areas in particular:[6]

➤ Robust selection processes

➤ Formal on-boarding of new staff

➤ Opportunities for promotion/advancement and new knowledge

[5] Howard, Ann; Debra Walker; Scott Erker; and Neal Bruce. "Feeling the Pain of Health Care's War for Talent." Selection Forecast 2006/07, pp. 1–17. Online white paper. www.ddiworld.com. Accessed 11/12/2010.
[6] Ibid.

The first two items on this list, robust selection and formal on-boarding of staff, were discussed in Chapter 18, Grow, Hire, Share, or Outsource. Mentoring is a form of intangible reward that can be provided to staff to assist with advancement and promotion; it is one way to meet the third retention strategy advocated by the experts.

A mentor assists an employee in planning his or her future trajectory and in working through issues and challenges. As important as mentoring is, we often do not see it actively used in medical practices. This is an oversight. A mentoring program in a medical practice cannot only help grow apprentice employees to become more than they even thought possible, but it also builds loyalty and employee engagement.

Similarly, a reverse mentoring program, where a more senior staff member calls on a more junior staffer to serve as a mentor, is also valuable in a medical practice. For example, a junior staffer who is well versed in social media can mentor the senior staff on correct Website design and design of social networking sites. This person can also be asked to educate senior staff on marketing techniques to target a specific patient cohort. These are just some examples of areas where reverse mentoring can benefit the senior staff and the medical practice, while at the same time permitting a junior staffer to shine and make a difference.

> Medical practices need to plan, implement, and manage the intangible rewards in a medical practice at the same or even greater level they give to their tangible and monetary rewards.

Intangible rewards often fall into one of three categories: recognition, celebration, and culture.[7] Examples of these types of intangible

---

[7] Walker, Deborah L. 1999. "Staff motivation and incentive plan development." *Journal of Medical Practice Management.* Nov/Dec 15(3):122–126.

rewards are provided in Exhibit 20.3.[8] Note that many of these have a strong impact, yet do not have a direct financial cost to the medical practice. For example, changing a job title may have a lot of meaning to a staff member, yet does not need to be accompanied by a salary increase for it to be effective in enhancing recognition of the employee's contribution to the medical practice. Medical practices need to plan, implement, and manage the intangible rewards in a medical practice at the same or even greater level they give to their tangible and monetary rewards.

| EXHIBIT 20.3 | Intangible Rewards |

Category	Activity
Recognition	➤ Praise
	➤ Changing a staff member's job title
	➤ Mentor programs
Celebration	➤ Social events
	➤ Seasonal events
Culture	➤ Active staff participation
	➤ Staff treated as professionals

Benefits

We leave a full discussion of employee benefits to the experts. However, two newer approaches to benefit design are worthy of comment.

Paid Time Off

Many medical practices have combined their separate time-off pools for sick leave, vacation, and holidays to form one paid-time-off

---

[8] For more ideas, see *1001 Ways to Reward Employees* by Bob Nelson (New York: Workman Publishers, 2005). Also, "Business owners try to motivate employees," by Sara E. Needleman (*Wall Street Journal*, Jan. 14, 2010, p. B-5).

(PTO) pool. In this fashion, the staff member is not placed into a position of having to manage each of these three "buckets" separately, recognizing that some staff need more sick leave, while others seek more vacation time.

A variation on the PTO model is to permit staff to donate some of their time to a colleague in need. For example, a staff member who has run out of PTO may be given 10 hours from a colleague's PTO bank to avoid taking leave without pay. Some medical practices take a simplistic view and provide the recipient with the donated hours, regardless of the wage level of the donor employee in comparison to the recipient. Other medical practices take a more complex approach, calculating the value of the PTO time and taking into consideration the comparative wage levels of the two parties. For example, an employee who makes $10 per hour and donates eight hours is donating a value of $80 to the recipient. In this situation, the $80 is divided by the recipient's hourly rate to result in the number of hours available for the recipient's use.

This sharing of PTO often enhances productivity in the medical practice. Studies have shown that "presenteeism" is costing employers more than absenteeism.[9] Presenteeism is when employees come to work ill and/or otherwise are not able to give 100 percent to the job. By permitting PTO to be shared with other members of the team, employees who are ill may stay at home rather than infect their colleagues (or patients) in the medical practice, which has a ripple effect in terms of lost productivity in the medical practice. Recipients of such donated time often report higher loyalty to and engagement in the medical practice and are appreciative of the team support.

Lifestyle Plans

Some medical practices have recognized that benefits that are valuable to one employee may not be relevant to another. They permit employees to select from a menu of benefit options (and have crafted

---

[9] Sitter, Daniel. "Presenteeism: The hidden costs of business." E-zine article. http://EzineArticles.com/?expert=Daniel_Sitter. Accessed 8/24/10.

these options in a legally compliant fashion). This permits employees to craft their benefit plans consistent with their personal needs rather than taking a one-size-fits-all approach. Lifestyle benefit plans are similar to the plans offered by payers that permit subscribers to mix and match premium levels, copayments, co-insurance, and deductibles, along with coverage levels when determining health insurance that is right for them and their families.

Distinguish Your Medical Practice

Two ways to distinguish your practice from other medical practices in the market are worthy of discussion.

Vacation Levels. As a recruiting aid, some medical practices not only offer competitive wage rates, but they also offer three weeks of vacation for starting employees (when the more typical vacation offering is two weeks). This extra week of vacation is not a direct out-of-pocket expense, yet it is a great incentive for an applicant to choose your medical practice over others. It also enforces the perception that you treat employees as professionals (which, of course, they are).

Expanded Roles and Compensation. A second distinguishing approach is to terminate the under-performing staff and ask the high performers to take on more responsibilities at a higher salary. A pediatrician shared the following example of this approach. Two under-performing employees were let go. A meeting was held with the three remaining staff, with the physician indicating that he believed these remaining staff were the best and the brightest of his staff. He indicated he has two options: recruit to replace the two staff members who were let go, or delegate additional roles and responsibilities to the remaining staff and increase their salaries by distributing the wages of the departing staff to them. The staff elected the higher salary and higher level of engagement with the medical practice. It actually cost the medical practice less money (due to savings on benefit expenditures), and it helped build a professional care team fully invested in the medical practice.

SUMMARY

In this chapter, we presented the key components of staff compensation and provided a variety of incentive plans for consideration by a medical practice. A combination of tangible and intangible rewards is needed in today's medical practices as we work to create a positive, energizing culture that is in a state of perpetual change and improvement.

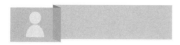

Conclusion

Your care team is the core competency of your medical practice. Its ability to work together, to innovate, and to make a difference in patients' lives is what truly distinguishes one medical practice from the next. In this book, we presented innovative staffing strategies so that you can bring your medical practice to the next level of performance. It is in the service to others — the purpose of our work in healthcare — that we truly become our very "best selves."

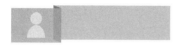

Q & A with Deborah Walker Keegan

WHY IS IT SO IMPORTANT TO GET STAFFING RIGHT?

Staff are the infrastructure and support for physician productivity. The physician's time is the limiting factor in a medical practice and it cannot be inventoried. Experts suggest that up to 60 percent of the physician's time is wasted. Thus, having the right staff doing the rights things is important in order to leverage the physician's time. A practice that has too few staff negatively impacts physician efficiency and practice profitability. At the same time, a practice that has too many staff has a higher staff overhead cost than other practices and is therefore less profitable. In addition, the staff impact the practice's ability to be efficient. With 80 to 85 percent of the cost of a medical practice "fixed," practice efficiency is now more important than ever as we work to reduce per-unit costs. Beyond productivity and cost implications, staff are important to enable quality patient care in a safe environment.

WHY DO WE NEED TO CHANGE OUR STAFFING MODEL OVER TIME?

It is important to recognize that staffing the medical practice is a continuous process — the work in a medical practice changes over time. The staffing deployment model should be reevaluated quarterly to make sure it is optimal. This should become a natural step that involves reassessing the resources in the practice to support patient care and physician productivity and efficiency.

Staffing is a measure of work. As the work levels and type of work in a practice change, the staffing model also needs to change, including staffing levels, skill mix, work processes, and work functions.

We now have three patient flow processes that need to be staffed with aligned staffing strategies — the internal patient flow process, which is the face-to-face visit; the external patient flow process, which is the telephones; and the virtual patient flow process, which is the Web portal, e-visits, secure message threads with patients, and other electronic patient access channels. Today's medical practice and its staffing needs are quite different from yesterday — and tomorrow's medical practice will present even more challenges.

HOW DO STAFF LEVELS AFFECT PROFITABILITY?

In a traditional medical practice that is reimbursed on a fee-for-service basis, profitability depends on the ability to streamline patient flow processes to permit high patient visit volumes. Staff are a resource in the medical practice to permit this streamlined patient flow, not simply a cost of doing business. In newer models of care, such as the medical home model, staff are a vital part of the care team. The entire care team is responsible for the value (defined as high quality at low cost) for an entire patient population.

When you analyze your staffing model, you may need more staff or a different skill mix of staff to support physicians and patients. Data suggest that better-performing medical practices with higher physician productivity actually have more staff. However, the cost of staff as a percentage of total medical revenue (which is the overhead cost attributed to staff) is lower, suggesting that these practices have the right staff doing the right things to support physicians in the medical practice.

WHY IS STAFFING DIFFERENT FROM PRACTICE TO PRACTICE, EVEN IN THE SAME SPECIALTY?

Staffing is practice specific because facility layout, physician productivity, technology leverage, multitasking of staff, type of practice, work delegation, and work processes and tools provided to the staff all influence the staffing needs of a medical practice. For example, a practice that has highly encumbered work processes needs more staff than one that has streamlined its processes. As another example, if physicians are highly productive, more staff are needed than in a medical practice with a low level of physician productivity. The actual work volume, type of work tasked to the staff, and the tools provided to the staff to perform their work dictate the staffing model specific to a medical practice.

HOW CAN STAFF PRODUCTIVITY BE TRACKED?

It is difficult to measure productivity of knowledge workers. One way to track staff productivity is to use expected staff workload ranges. We use these ranges to determine if there is opportunity to redesign the staffing model of a medical practice. For example, one staff member working full time can typically check in approximately 70 patients at the front desk. The work of the current staff can be analyzed and compared to this level. The performance workload range for a particular practice can be identified by watching the staff perform their work and identifying the typical amount of time it takes to perform a task. But it is important to recognize that quality needs to trump quantity. If the staff cannot perform high-quality work, you may need to relax the volume expectations for the work. Staff are not robots, and the work required of a medical practice is knowledge work, which cannot be measured simply on work quantity alone.

WHAT ARE THE BEST REWARDS TO USE IN A MEDICAL PRACTICE?

In addition to offering higher wage rates than competing practices, experienced employees can be valued by delegating real responsibility to them. For example, an experienced staff member can be asked to investigate the latest scheduling techniques and become the team expert, suggesting changes and educating other staff. By expecting more in terms of talent and contribution, we demonstrate the value of staff — and rely on staff — as partners in the care team.

Nontangible rewards such as recognition and flexible work schedules are more important than financial incentives to many employees. Treating staff as the professionals that they are and ensuring that their work is directly connected to the patient are vital to the care team approach to patient service delivery that we seek.

WHAT DO YOU THINK ARE THE CRITICAL ELEMENTS TO STAFFING THE MEDICAL PRACTICE?

The callouts in each chapter summarize many of the critical elements to innovative staffing of the medical practice. These are restated below.

Chapter 1: Optimal Staffing of the Medical Practice: An Overview

Indeed, the only true value-added steps in the entire patient flow process from the patient's point of view is the actual time the patient spends in the exam room with the physician or when receiving care via virtual medicine.

Service is often considered a proxy for quality. Thus, if service is suboptimal, patients will often interpret this to mean that quality, too, is below par.

One of the toughest challenges for any medical practice is to ratchet up productivity once staff are used to working at a certain pace.

In addition to staffing the face-to-face visit and the telephones, we need to staff for virtual medicine. The Web portal, virtual visits with providers, care and case management, health coaching and outreach, and secure message threads with the care team require a distinct focus of staff roles and responsibilities.

Chapter 2: Staff for the Future Now

Today's medical practices are expanding patient access channels to ensure that patients are engaged and active in their care.

The work of ensuring that the patient's care and treatment are consistent with evidence-based guidelines and established targets and goals rests with the provider and clinical support staff, necessitating a change to their work scope and effort.

Medical practices that participate in risk-based reimbursement need to assign staff to support the patient visit and the medical practice in new ways in order to support the physicians and achieve financial success.

Chapter 3: How to Analyze Your Staffing Deployment Model

A staffing deployment model is the model that describes your staff and their assigned roles and responsibilities.

Over time, the medical practice has grown or expanded or changed, while the staffing model remained unchanged and is no longer current.

By arraying your staffing deployment model and asking key questions, you begin to understand potential opportunities to improve the infrastructure and support to the physician and patient.

Chapter 4: The Staff Benchmarking Process

The impact on profitability is not necessarily the result of having more staff but rather of having the right staff doing the right things that are contributing to practice profitability.

There are limitations to the benchmark data. Despite these limitations, benchmarking staff levels and costs to peer practices helps to identify opportunities for improvement.

Chapter 5: The Staff Workload Evaluation Process

There are different staff workload ranges depending on the type of work that has been delegated to the staff to perform.

Staff are not robots, and day-to-date practice operations are not always routine. Quality needs to trump quantity each and every time.

By comparing actual work levels, you are in a better position to determine whether you have the right number of staff devoted to a particular work function and task.

Chapter 6: Creating a Care Team

Imagine a new staffing strategy with the patient at the center of the care team.

In essence, we want the team to "become who we are" not "what we want to be."

Share as much financial and operational information as possible with your team.

Through these actions, you begin to transition staff from employee to partner, one who has a sense of ownership and pride in the work and work product and makes a true contribution to the team.

Chapter 7: Staffing the Telephones

The traditional call management process for a medical practice is costly and encumbered.

We recommend that the work of telephone management be separated from the work of the face-to-face visit with the patient.

The most innovative process for telephone management is to replace the telephone with online patient access.

Chapter 8: Staffing the Front Office

The front office staff largely determine whether or not a clean claim is submitted to payers.

The front office staff serve as marketers, billers, information processors, reimbursement managers, and a host of other roles.

Eliminate waiting and queuing and bring the work to the patient. Consider eliminating the check-in and check-out desks and conduct this work in the exam room.

Chapter 9: Staffing the Visit

Clinical staff who support the patient visit and patient flow should be up on their feet anticipating both physician and patient needs and actively participating in the actual patient visit.

The most efficient organization of nurse triage and advice staff is to co-locate these staff to permit resource sharing and knowledge support.

It is not physically possible for a single nurse to provide patient flow and visit support 25 to 30 patient visits and also manage 100 to 120 telephone calls in a timely and accurate fashion. Identify clinical staff to manage patient flow and visit support and separate clinical staff to manage telephone calls and virtual medicine.

Chapter 10: Staffing the Billing Office

For front-end billing, staff based at the practice site need payer-specific knowledge so they can manage patient financial clearance, conduct accurate registration, obtain waiver forms, and collect time-of-service payments.

Staffing the revenue cycle of the future will largely rest with staff at the practice sites and with staff located in proximity to where the patient receives care.

Chapter 11: Staffing for Medical Records and Electronic Health Records

With EHRs, a redesign of the patient flow process is needed to expand patient access and communication options. This requires a dramatic change to the current staffing deployment model of a medical practice.

When EHRs are introduced in a medical practice, the physician's inbox is like a living, breathing appendage. Staff need to be deployed to assist with this work.

It is important to recognize that with EHRs, the patient visit does not need to continue to consist of a set of sequential steps.

Chapter 12: Staffing the Medical Home Model

In a medical home model, patients are assigned to a personal care physician, and the physician and care team provide access and outreach to the patient on a 24/7 basis.

Coordination of care is facilitated by clinical information systems, registries, telehealth, and other modalities to ensure timely and appropriate care for the patient.

The organizations that have demonstrated success with medical home models have a heightened involvement of clinical support staff. In addition, patients in medical homes appear to be more actively engaged in their care.

Chapter 13: Staffing Models for Fluctuating Work Levels and Other Realities

With fluctuating patient visit volume, a static staffing model means that the medical practice will either overstaff or understaff for the work.

Part-time staff fill the void and create the "step-up" assistance that is needed.

The dual-shift model of care and its associated staffing pattern increases facility utilization and spreads the cost over more patients, thereby reducing cost per visit.

Chapter 14: Part-Time Staff and Virtual Staff

With part-time staff on board, the medical practice can achieve productivity gains and also meet patient expectations for service in a way that is difficult for the full-time staff member who is trying to play catch-up at the end of a busy week.

Student interns are another source of part-time staff. These students often have a vested interest in performing well and can be a valuable addition to the care team.

Medical practices that previously relied on temporary agencies are increasingly recognizing the need to develop internal part-time staff or float pools with staff fully trained to the systems and technology.

Advances in technology permit virtual employees to participate in collective forums, such as meetings, while conducting their work from home (or, in actuality, from wherever they have the required access to technology).

Chapter 15: Role Options for Nonphysician Providers

There are two primary roles nonphysician providers play in a medical practice: leverage and production.

In some settings, physicians compete with the nurse practitioner or physician assistant for patients, which is an unintended consequence of the provider model.

With a shortage of physicians in many markets, a rotational model involving the physician and nonphysicain provider is prevalent.

In many medical practices, it is evident that the nonphysician provider model has evolved over time rather than being formed with a clear and distinct strategy.

Chapter 16: Work Process Redesign

Lean serves as a galvanizing force to overcome inertia to change, and it serves as a catalyst to create a new organizational culture.

In a typical day, we have "time creep." Time simply flies by, and it is very difficult to ensure that all the required functions and tasks are attended to.

By expecting the huddle to be held and the formal agenda to be followed, medical practice leaders ensure that the work will be performed in a standard, systematic, and efficient manner — each time, every time.

Everyone is expected to do the same work and perform the same process steps, with the same timelines. Importantly, this is done each time, every time.

Chapter 17: Creating Purposeful Work

You do meaningful work each and every day. This purpose stimulates employee commitment and creativity.

To truly engage staff members in the work of a medical practice, it is important for them to actually connect their work and effort to the patient.

The knowledge workers in our medical practices are dual-focus workers.

Chapter 18: Grow, Hire, Share, or Outsource

When a medical practice has a staff vacancy, it is an opportune time to revisit the staffing model. It may be that a new staff member is not needed if a change is made to the existing staffing deployment model.

New employees need to possess the intellectual capital to do the work, as well as the relational and social capital to work in a care team providing service to patients.

Focus on selective recruiting — identifying individuals with skill, talent, and a cultural and value fit with the medical practice.

Chapter 19: Talent Management: Nurse Betty Behaving Badly

The real question we should be asking about these staff is, are they adding value to the practice?

The key to talent management is holding individuals accountable for performance and results.

The manager's role is to ensure that the staff have the tools and support needed for them to exercise their strengths.

Chapter 20: Staff Compensation and Incentive Plans

The challenge in knowledge work is to determine how to best measure productivity.

In today's medical practices, there is a shift away from permanent increases to the base salary due to the financial model of many medical practices and the uncertainty regarding payer reimbursement.

By carefully crafting an incentive plan for your medical practice, you can work to avoid unintended consequences.

Medical practices need to plan, implement, and manage the intangible rewards in a medical practice at the same or even greater level they give to their tangible and monetary rewards.

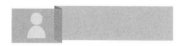

Additional Resources

This list of resources has been compiled for your reference and does not represent our commercial endorsement of any particular product or association. You may want to investigate these and other resources as you innovate the staffing deployment model of your medical practice.

LEADERSHIP AND MANAGEMENT

Drucker, Peter F. 1973. *Management: Tasks, Responsibilities, and Practices*. New York: HarperBusiness.

Drucker, Peter F. 1990. *Managing the Nonprofit Organization: Principles and Practices*. New York: Collins Business.

Drucker, Peter F. 2004. *The Daily Drucker: 366 Days of Insight and Motivation for Getting the Right Things Done*. New York: HarperBusiness.

Edersheim, Elizabeth H. 2007. *The Definitive Drucker*. New York: McGraw-Hill.

Ellsworth, Richard R. 2002. *Leading with Purpose: The New Corporate Realities*. Stanford, Calif.: Stanford Business Books.

Goleman, Daniel. 1995. *Emotional Intelligence: Why It Can Matter More than IQ*. New York: Bantam Books.

LEAN MANAGEMENT SYSTEMS

Black, John, with David Miller. 2008. *The Toyota Way to Healthcare Excellence: Increase Efficiency and Improve Quality with Lean*. Chicago: Health Administration Press.

Womack, James P., and Daniel T. Jones. 2008. *Lean Thinking: Banish Waste and Create Wealth in Your Corporation*. London: Simon and Schuster.

MEDICAL HOME MODEL

Johns Hopkins University. Guided Care. www.guidedcare.org.

Kuzel, Anton J. 2009. "Ten steps to a patient-centered medical home." *Fam Pract Manag*. www.aafp.org/online/en/home/publications/journals/fpm/preprint/kuzel.printerviewhtml/. Accessed 1/23/10.

National Center for Medical Home Implementation. www.medicalhomeinfo.org.

Patient-Centered Primary Care Collaborative. www.pcpcc.net.

Reid, Robert, J.; Katie Coleman; Eric A. Johnson; "The group health medical home at year two: Cost savings, higher patient satisfaction and less burnout for physicians." *Health Affairs*. 29(5):835–843.

TransforMed. www.transformed.com.

STAFF BENCHMARKING*

Medical Group Management Association. *Cost Survey for Multispecialty Practices*. Englewood, Colo.: Medical Group Management Association.

Medical Group Management Association. *Cost Survey for Single-Specialty Practices*. Englewood, Colo.: Medical Group Management Association.

Medical Group Management Association. *Performance and Practices of Successful Medical Groups*. Englewood, Colo.: Medical Group Management Association.

These survey reports are published annually.

STAFF COMPENSATION

The Health Care Group, Inc. Staff Salary Survey.
www.healthcaregroup.com.

Johnson, Bruce, and Deborah Walker Keegan. 2006. *Physician Compensation Plans: State-of-the-Art Strategies*. Englewood, Colo.: Medical Group Management Association.

Needleman, Sara E. 2010. "Business owners try to motivate employees." *Wall Street Journal*. Jan. 14, p. B-5.

Nelson, Bob. 2005. *1001 Ways to Reward Employees*. New York: Workman Publishers.

Schumpeter. 2002. "Overstretched. Many people who keep their jobs are working too hard. What can companies do about it?" *The Economist*. Business Section, May 22, p. 72.

Professional Association of Health Care Office Management (PAHCOM) Annual Salary Survey. www.pahcom.com.

Salary Wizard. www.salary.com.

Spolsky, Joel. "Why I never let employees negotiate pay raises." *Software, Inc*. April 2009, pp. 37–38.

Walker, Deborah L. 1999. "Staff motivation and incentive plan development." *Journal of Medical Practice Management*. Nov/Dec 15(3):122–126.

STAFFING TOOLS AND STRATEGIES

Anderson, Benjamin, and John Rozich. 2001. "Your practice's most important 'work-in': Bringing certified nurse practitioners on to the treatment team." *MGMA Connexion*. 1(1):60–65.

Anderson, Peter, and Marc D. Halley. 2008 "A new approach to making your doctor–nurse team more productive." *Fam Pract Manag*. 15(17):35–40.

Bernthal, Paul, and James Davis. Monograph. *Service Skills in the Workplace*. Development Dimensions International, Inc. Revised MMIV, pp. 1–28. www.ddiworld.com. Accessed 11/09/10.

Bernthal, Paul. Executive Summary. *Recruitment and Selection.* Developmental Dimensions International, Inc. Revised MMII, pp. 1–20.

Burlingham, Bo. "In times like these you get a chance to show your strength," Interview with Jim Collins. *Inc. Magazine,* April 2009, p. 81.

Burud, Sandra, and Marie Tumolo. 2004. *Leveraging the New Human Capital: Adaptive Strategies, Results Achieved, and Stories of Transformation.* Palo Alto, Calif.: Davies-Black Publishing.

Davidson, Paul. "Contract workers swelling ranks." *USA Today.* Money Section. Dec. 2, 2009, p. B-1.

Family Team Care. www.familyteamcare.org

Healthcare Intelligence Network. 2010 Health Coaching Benchmarks: Operations and Performance Data for Optimal Program ROI and Participant Health Status. Based on 2009 HIN Health & Wellness Coaching Survey. www.him.com and www.hin.com/chartoftheweek/health_coaching_monthly_caseload. Accessed 11/10/2010.

Howard, Ann, Debra Walker, Scott Erker, and Neal Bruce. Feeling the Pain of Health Care's War for Talent. Selection Forecast 2006/07. pp. 1–17. Online white paper. www.ddiworld.com. Accessed 11/12/2010.

Institute of Medicine. 2001. *Crossing the Quality Chasm: A New Health System for the 21st Century.* Washington, DC: National Academy Press.

Levoy, Bob. 2007. *222 Secrets of Hiring, Managing, and Retaining Great Employees in Healthcare Practices.* Sudbury, Mass.: Jones and Bartlett.

Magill, Michael K., Robin L. Lloyd, Duane Palmer, Susan A. Terry. 2006. "Successful turnaround of a university-owned, community-based, multidisciplinary practice network." *Ann Fam Med.* 4(Supplement 1):S19–21. www.annfammed.org. Accessed 11/11/2010.

Novak, Alys, and Courtney Price. 2007. *HR Policies & Procedures Manual for Medical Practices, 4th Edition*. Englewood, Colo.: Medical Group Management Association.

Novak, Alys, and Courtney Price. 2008. *Job Description Manual for Medical Practices, 3rd Edition*. Englewood, Colo.: Medical Group Management Association.

Oetjen, Reid M., and Dawn M. Oetjen. 2009. "Free labor! How to successfully use student interns in your practice." *J. Med. Pract. Manage.* 24(6):376–380.

Online Job Descriptions. O*Net Online. www.online.onetcenter.org.

Siehl, Caren, David E. Bowen, and Christine Pearson. 1992. Service encounters as rites of integration: An information processing model. *Organization Science.* 3(4):537–555.

Sitter, Daniel. "Presenteeism: The hidden costs of business." E-zine article. http://EzineArticles.com/?expert=Daniel_Sitter. Accessed 8/24/10.

Society for Human Resource Management (SHRM). www.shrm.org.

Walker Keegan, Deborah L.; Elizabeth W. Woodcock; and Sara M. Larch. 2009. *The Physician Billing Process: 12 Potholes to Avoid in the Road to Getting Paid*. Englewood, Colo.: Medical Group Management Association.

Woodcock, Elizabeth W. 2007. "Total account ownership: A new model for streamlining your business office staff. *MGMA Connexion.* 7(1):28–33.

Woodcock, Elizabeth W. 2009. *Mastering Patient Flow: Using Lean Thinking to Improve Your Practice Operations*. Englewood, Colo.: Medical Group Management Association.

Woodcock, Elizabeth W. 2011. *Front Office Success: How to Satisfy Patients and Boost the Bottom Line*. Englewood, Colo.: Medical Group Management Association.

Woodcock, Elizabeth W., and Bette A. Warn, 2011. *Operating Policies & Procedures Manual for Medical Practices, 4th Edition*. Englewood, Colo.: Medical Group Management Association.

TEAMS

Lencioni, Patrick. 2002. *The Five Dysfunctions of a Team: A Leadership Fable*. San Francisco: Jossey-Bass.

Walker, Deborah. 1999. "Laying the Foundation for Continual Change: Teaming for Innovation," in Key, M.K.: *Managing Change in Healthcare: Innovative Solutions for People-Based Organizations*. New York: McGraw-Hill.

Index

Note: *ex.* indicates exhibit.

About MGMA

MGMA is the premier membership association for professional administrators and leaders of medical group practices. Since 1926, MGMA has delivered networking, professional education and resources, and political advocacy for medical practice management. Today, MGMA's 22,500 members lead 13,600 organizations nationwide in which some 280,000 physicians provide more than 40 percent of the healthcare services delivered in the United States.

MGMA's mission is to continually improve the performance of medical group practice professionals and the organizations they represent. MGMA promotes the group practice model as the optimal framework for healthcare delivery, assisting group practices in providing efficient, safe, patient-focused, and affordable care.

MGMA is headquartered in Englewood, Colo., and maintains a government affairs office in Washington, D.C.

About ACMPE

Founded in 1956, ACMPE is the standard-setting and certification organization of MGMA. Through ACMPE, medical group managers can earn the Certified Medical Practice Executive (CMPE) designation and go on to earn the highest distinction of Fellow in the ACMPE (FACMPE). ACMPE members belong to a network of management professionals dedicated to becoming the best in medical practice management by combining experience, learning, and professional certification.

MGMA STAFFING TOOL

www.mgma.com/innovativestaffing

This Web link connects you to an *annually* updated staff modeling tool that allows you to input your staffing data and compare it to the most recent MGMA median benchmarks. In turn, you may identify opportunities to improve staffing and practice performance.